Legg-Calvé-Perthes' Disease

CURRENT PROBLEMS IN ORTHOPAEDICS

This series of monographs, each written or edited by a distinguished authority, deals with special topics in orthopaedics, particularly those which present major problems in diagnosis and management, and where recent research advances carry important implications for patient care.

Editorial Advisory Board

Richard Cruess, Montreal
Henry Mankin, Boston
Brian McKibbin, Cardiff
Michael Freeman, London
Alf Nachemson, Göteborg
Marvin Tile, Toronto

Already published

Menelaus: The Orthopaedic Management of Spina Bifida Cystica, 2ed
Sevitt: Bone Repair and Fracture Healing in Man
Dandy: Arthroscopic Surgery of the Knee
Turco: Club Foot

In preparation

Leffert: The Brachial Plexus
Ling: Complications of Total Hip Replacement
Galasko: Radionuclide Scintigraphy in Orthopaedics
Samuelson & Freeman: Surgical Treatment of the Arthritic Ankle and Foot

Legg-Calvé-Perthes' Disease

Anthony Catterall MChir FRCS
Consultant Orthopaedic Surgeon,
Royal National Orthopaedic Hospital and Charing Cross
Hospital, London

Foreword by
G.C. Lloyd-Roberts MChir FRCS
Honorary Orthopaedic Surgeon, Hospital for Sick Children
and St George's Hospital, London

CHURCHILL LIVINGSTONE
EDINBURGH LONDON MELBOURNE AND NEW YORK 1982

CHURCHILL LIVINGSTONE
Medical Division of Longman Group Limited

Distributed in the United States of America by Churchill
Livingstone Inc., 19 West 44th Street, New York, N.Y.
10036, and by associated companies, branches and
representatives throughout the world.

First published 1982

ISBN 0 443 01942 8

British Library Cataloguing in Publication Data
Catterall, Anthony
    Legg-Calvé-Perthes' disease. — (Current problems in
    orthopaedics)
    1. Hip joint — Diseases 2. Children — Diseases
    I. Title   II. Series
    617'.581   RJ480

Library of Congress Catalog Card Number 81–68934

Printed in Great Britain by
William Clowes (Beccles) Limited, Beccles and London

Foreword

In recent years notable progress has been made in our understanding of the aetiology, natural history and histopathology of Legg-Calvé-Perthes' disease. As a result our concepts of management have inevitably required re-appraisal — a process which continues to evolve. So rapid a development of knowledge rightly fosters uncertainty and controversy and it is fortunate, therefore, that a monograph devoted to this disorder should appear at this time. It is, however, essential that the source be authoritative and it is, therefore, doubly fortunate that the author of this work has made important contributions to almost every facet of our recently acquired and still expanding knowledge.

This book commends itself by virtue of this authority which thereby renders further commendation, however sincere, superfluous.

G.C.L.-R.

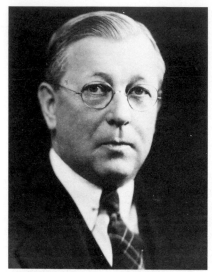

Arthur T. Legg
1874–1939

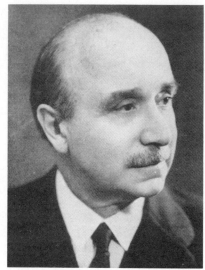

Jacques Calvé
1875–1954

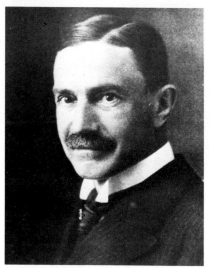

Georg Perthes
1869–1927

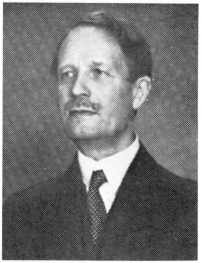

Henning Waldenström
1877–1972

Preface

Seventy years ago the reports by Legg, Calvé and Perthes identified a non-tuberculous condition of the child's hip leading to osteoarthritis in the adult. At this time the major causes of crippling disease were poliomyelitis, chronic infection and arthritis. The literature, therefore, reflected the magnitude of these problems. As the result of much research vaccination has largely eliminated poliomyelitis; antibiotics, the problems related to chronic infection; and joint replacement, the pain and disability of arthritis. Despite much research into the aetiology, pathology and methods of treatment the cause of Legg-Calvé-Perthes' disease remains unresolved, and the treatment therefore empirical. Because of this the literature continues to blossom with reports in which scientific facts are often few and controversial theory freely discussed.

Why, then, should another book be added to this subject when the literature is already so extensive?

There is need with any problem about which much is written for a periodic review of the subject in general, with presentation of new material. The reviews by Goff (1954) and Edgren (1965) have in the past admirably met this need and it is hoped that the present contribution will meet this requirement in both of its aspects.

I felt that it was unnecessary when writing this book to review in detail all the theories and contributions discussed by these authors, but to highlight points in all aspects of this condition in which changes are occurring and to support these views from the historical literature and from data that I have been able to collect personally.

With these thoughts in mind the book is laid out in a number of chapters, all of which are providing evidence to a central hypothesis, which is stated in the first chapter and reviewed in the final one. Whether or not this hypothesis will stand the test of time must be the subject of further research and reports but the evidence as laid out in this book has encouraged me to go forward. .

Criticism has recently been made that the radiological classification that I suggested some years ago has proved difficult to use in clinical practice because of difficulty in the assessment of the radiographs. The chapter on radiological features has taken note of this problem and tried to clarify the radiological criteria on which the diagnosis of Group and 'head-at-risk' signs are made. In collaboration with my colleagues at the Institute of Orthopaedics, and through the generosity of the authors of previous published reports, a careful study has been made of the morbid anatomy of this process by reviewing a total of four whole femoral heads. This gives some degree of understanding to the morbid anatomical features and their radiological appearances. On the basis of these two aspects a protocol is developed for treatment of these children and the results of a prospective series of treated cases reviewed. I am aware that even as a result of this study we are no nearer to the cause of this problem. I hope, however, that the thoughts which are laid out in this discussion may stimulate research which may eventually lead to a true understanding of the causative factors. If this objective is finally achieved then the endeavour of this book and others like it will have been worthwhile.

London, 1982   A.C.

To my wife

Acknowledgements

It is a great pleasure for me to acknowledge the considerable help, advice and support that I have received in the preparation of this monograph.

It was Mr G.C. Lloyd-Roberts who in 1968 initially stimulated my interest in this problem. He has supported and encouraged my research over the ensuing years and it is therefore a particular privilege for me that he has generously agreed to write the Foreword to this book.

It is through the generosity of Professor Dolman and Dr M. Bell, Professor B. McKibbin and Dr Z. Ralis, Dr I. Ponseti and Mr G. Fulford that I was able to bring together the morphological material which is reviewed in this book. This study would not have been possible without the help and guidance of my colleagues Dr J. Pringle, Dr P. Byers, Mr H.B.S. Kemp and the technical staff of the Department of Morbid Anatomy at the Institute of Orthopaedics, London.

Many orthopaedic surgeons have kindly referred cases of Legg-Calvé-Perthes' disease to me for treatment. Without these clinical cases it would not have been possible to develop the current thoughts on management. Mr W. Muirhead-Allwood and Mr G. Grossbard have generously reviewed the results of treatment of these cases and also the problems in adolescence. The important computer study of the 388 cases which formed the basis of the 1970 survey has been undertaken by Mr S. Wientroub.

I am particularly grateful to Miss U. Boundy and Mr Collins of the Department of Medical Photography at the Royal National Orthopaedic Hospital, London, and Miss M. Hudson and Mr R. Williams of the Department of Medical Illustration at the New Charing Cross Hospital, London, for the enormous labour of preparing the illustrations without which this monograph could not have been presented.

Obtaining the photographs of the 'four great men of the Legg-Calvé-Perthes' disease controversy' has proved extremely difficult. I am therefore very grateful to Dr Thornton Brown for obtaining the photograph of Dr A.T. Legg from the files of the *Journal of Bone and Joint Surgery* in Boston and to the Council of Management of the *Journal of Bone and Joint Surgery*, London, for permission to reproduce the photograph of Dr J. Calvé. Professor Tonnis generously located the photograph of Dr Georg Perthes and obtained permission for me to reproduce it. Professor Ian Goldie of Goteborg, Sweden, generously agreed to approach the Waldenström family to allow me to reproduce the photograph of Professor Henning Waldenström. I am also grateful to the Council of Management and Board of Trustees of the *Journal of Bone and Joint Surgery* for permission to reproduce Figures 3.6, 5.11, 5.15, 5.18, 5.21; to Mr A. Apley and Butterworths and Co., for permission to reproduce Figures 5.8, 5.10, 5.13, 5.16, 5.17 and to Dr Murray and Churchill Livingstone for permission to reproduce Figure 5.4.

Finally I am grateful to my wife who has not only supported this venture with her understanding and forbearance but also typed the text and tables.

A.C.

Contents

1. **The past and present** 1

2. **Aetiology** 3
   Incidence 3
   Inherited factors 3
   Epidemiological factors 4
   Constitutional factors 4
   Associated anomalies 5
   Conclusions 6

3. **Morbid anatomy** 8
   Historical review 8
   The anatomy of the normal femoral head
      in the child and the consequence of
      infarction 9
   Review of human case material 12
      (a) the uninvolved hip 12
      (b) involved femoral heads 13
      (c) metaphyseal changes 28
   Discussion of human case material 31

4. **Clinical features** 34
   Age and sex 34
   Bilateral cases 34
   Presentation — acute 35
      — chronic 36
   Follow-up examinations 37
   Investigation 37
      Bone scan 37

5. **Radiological features** 39
   Differential diagnosis of a Perthes-like
      change 39
   Radiological features of the irritable hip
      syndrome 43
   Legg-Calvé-Perthes' disease 43
      Early diagnosis 44
      The stages of the disease and its
         natural history 45

The extent of epiphyseal involve-
   ment (the Groups) 45
Results in untreated cases 57
Age and sex within the Groups 58
Metaphyseal changes 59
Duration of the disease 60
Radiological course and the signs of
   healing 61
Osteochondritis dissecans 61

6. **The long term prognosis** 65
   Historical review 65
   1970 review 65
   Radiological changes in the long term 69
   Conclusions 70

7. **The poor result** 71
   The mechanism of femoral head de-
      formity 71
   Radiological signs of deterioration in the
      shape of the femoral head 74
   The concept of the 'head-at-risk' 76
   Poor results in the long term 79
   Conclusions 79

8. **Treatment** 81
   The principles of treatment 82
   The new principles 83
   Assessment of end results 84
   The indications for treatment 84
   The potential for remaining growth 86
   Clinical assessment 88
   Examination under anaesthetic and
      arthrography 88
   Containment of the femoral head and
      mobilisation of the hip joint 91
   Maintenance of containment until head
      is established 92

8. Treatment (*contd*)
The technique of femoral osteotomy   95
The assessment of the late case   97

9. The results of treatment   101
Clinical material   101
Methods of treatment   101

Results of treatment   102
Conclusions   106

10. The future   110

Index   113

1

The past and present

With the discovery of X-rays by Röntgen in 1895 the stage was set for improvement in diagnosis and treatment throughout the fields of medicine. Particularly in orthopaedics, the images produced by these X-rays allowed a more precise diagnosis of many conditions which had previously been lumped together under the broad headings of chronic infection, fracture and arthritis. It had been realised since the early 1900s (Hoffa 1903, Frieberg 1905) that there were conditions in the child and adolescent which lead to Osteoarthritis Deformans in the adult. However, the clear delineation of the condition which we now call Legg-Calvé-Perthes' disease or Coxa Plana was not made until 1909 and 1910.

There is some confusion as to the historical details and timing of these reports because, although five people published closely related descriptions of this topic, only three recognised that it was non-tuberculous.

The diary of these events is described by Sundt (1920). In 1909 Waldenström described this condition, regarding it as a benign form of tuberculosis, and later in the same year Legg read his famous paper at a Meeting of the American Orthopaedic Association in Hartford, while Sourdat published a thesis on the radiological features of the painful hip in children. The following year, 1910, the now classical papers by Calvé, Legg and Perthes were published; each individually describing a deformity of the growing hip in children. In 1913 Perthes wrote his second article, introducing the name Osteochondritis Deformans Juvenilis to describe this entity and implying that this was primarily an osteochondritis. In 1916 Legg published a formal review of many of the previously reported

cases. He concluded that some but not all of the cases reported by Waldenström and Sourdat in 1909 should be included as the descriptions of this condition. He also stated 'A new clinical entity has emerged in the category of a juvenile disease affecting the hip. This is largely due to the work of Dr Georg Perthes, who, after a preliminary study in 1910, both clinical in his own cases and bibliographical in the prior reports, in 1913 presented a classical monograph on the affection in question'. It is largely due to this paper that the title Perthes' disease came to be used by many orthopaedic surgeons in the British Isles when considering this condition. In 1920 Waldenström, Perthes, and Sundt published articles in *Zéntralblatt fur Chirurgie*. The paper by Waldenström introduces the name Coxa Plana to the literature. He regarded this term as useful in that it implied neither aetiology nor outcome. This name, which has also been used by many surgeons throughout the world, also underlines much of the controversy that exists in a condition where even the title cannot be agreed upon by those interested in it. Because the cause of this condition remains obscure the literature has blossomed and the pendulum of change, particularly with regard to treatment, has provided orthopaedic surgeons with controversy for debate in learned societies and orthopaedic books of reference.

The chapters of this book will consider in detail the present knowledge of all aspects of this problem. This information is derived from historical reports in the literature and from observations that I have been able to make personally. I would like to suggest to the reader that as he reviews the evidence presented he should consider it in terms of a working hypothesis. This hypothesis would state that:

 In the susceptible child the changes which are called Legg-Calvé-Perthes' disease are the consequence of ischaemia of variable duration, after which the process of repair produces a growth disturbance, which if uncontrolled leads to femoral head deformity with subsequent arthritis.

REFERENCES

Calvé J 1910 Sur une forme particulare de pseudo-coxalgia greffee sur des deformations caracteristiques de l'extremite superiure due femur. Revue de Chirurgie 30: 54–84

Frieberg A H 1905 Coxa vara adolescentrium and osteoarthritis deformans coxae. American Journal of Orthopaedic Surgery 1905

Hoffa A 1903 Quoted by Legg A T 1916. Osteochondral trophopathy of the hip joint. Surgery, Gynaecology and Obstetrics 22: 307–323

Legg A T 1910 An obscure affection of the hip joint. Boston Medical and Surgical Journal 162; 202–204

Legg A T 1916 Osteochondral trophopathy of the hip joint. Surgery, Gynaecology and Obstetrics 22: 307–323

Perthes G C 1910 Uber arthritis deformans juvenilis. Deutsche Zeitschrift fur Chirurgie 107: 11–59

Perthes G C 1913 Osteochondritis deformans juvenilis. Archives fur Klinishche Chirurgie 101: 779–807

Perthes G 1920 Beitrag zur atiologie der osteochondirits deformans, nebst Bemerkungen zu den artikel von Sundt und Con Waldenstrom. Zentralblatt fur Chirurgie 47: 542–547

Sourdat P 1909 Etude radiographiquie de al hanche coxalgique – Thesis Paris 1909 quoted by Edgren W Acta Orthopaedica Scandinavica Suppl 84: 14

Sundt H 1920 Malum coxae Calve-Legg-Perthes. Zentralblatt fur Chirurgie 47: 538–539

Waldenström H 1909 Der obere tuberkulose collumherd. Zeitschrift fur Orthopadische Chirurgie 24: 487–512

Waldenström H 1920 Coxa plana, osteochondritis deformans coxae, Calve-Perthessche Krankheit, Legg disease. Zentralblatt fur Chirurgie 47: 539–542

Aetiology

Despite an increasing volume of literature the cause of this condition remains obscure. It is now generally accepted that the major underlying process is that of avascular necrosis of the upper femoral epiphysis. This follows the demonstration of necrotic bone within the substance of the epiphysis by Phemister in 1921. Many theories have been advanced to explain this necrosis and the subsequent changes. Amongst these are trauma, inflammation secondary to bacterial infection, endocrine and nutritional causes, and circulatory abnormalities including micotic embolism. These theories are reviewed in the excellent monograph by Edgren (1965). Although each of these may on occasion be used to explain the cause of Legg-Calvé-Perthes' disease the aetiology in the majority remains unknown. It is logical, therefore, to consider the evidence that has been presented and to see if conclusions may be drawn to support the idea that there is a susceptible child in whom this disease may occur.

Table 2.1 Incidence of Legg-Calvé-Perthes' disease in various parts of the world.

Source	Area	Overall	Boys	Girls
Molloy 1966	Massachusetts	1:1200	1:740	1:3700
Helbo 1953	Denmark	1:2300		
Gray 1972	British Columbia	1:1400	1:820	1:4500

Table 2.2 Incidence of Legg-Calvé-Perthes' disease in the British Isles.

Source	Area	Overall	Boys	Girls
Harper 1976	South Wales	1:4750	1:3000	1:11 800
Catterall 1970	Scotland	1:5590	1:4060	1:14 830
Barker 1980	England	1:12 500	1:8064	1:30 300
	Merseyside		1:5917	1:20 000
	Trent		1:8333	1:33 000
	Wessex		1:11 494	1:50 000

Incidence

It is difficult to be sure of the true incidence of this condition as many cases escape undiagnosed, only to present late in adult life with secondary osteoarthritis of the hip which is the late manifestation of this disease. Tables 2.1 and 2.2 set out the recorded instances in several parts of the world. Although showing differences they are all approximately of the same order of magnitude and therefore probably represent an overall incidence of this condition. The recent paper by Barker (1978) is of interest in that for the first time it shows a regional variation of this condition with a higher incidence in towns than in rural communities. This may represent a difference in the environment of these children; those in towns play in playgrounds while those in the country play in the garden. It may also represent a change in social class as has been emphasised by Wynne-Davies and Gormley (1978). I have investigated the incidence in Scotland and found similar figures to those on Merseyside. It was not possible to investigate a regional incidence with the data available.

Inherited factors

It is reported that the incidence of Perthes' disease in families is greater than that of the general population. In many cases, however, a strong family history, particularly of bilateral disease, is more suggestive of one of the skeletal dypslasias of which multiple epiphyseal dysplasia and spondylo-epiphyseal dysplasia are typical examples and must be carefully excluded in the assessment of any suspected case of Legg-Calvé-Perthes' disease. Where these conditions have been eliminated it has usually been found that the incidence of disease in the first degree relatives is low (Wansbrough et al 1959, Gray et al 1972, Fisher 1972, Wynne-Davies and Gormley 1978). In the recent survey by Wynne-Davies and Gormley the definite conclusion has been reached that there are no inherited factors in this process. The evidence is suggestive for the following reasons:

1. The frequency amongst first degree relatives is low.
2. The frequency amongst second and third degree relatives approaches that of the normal population.
3. If Legg-Calvé-Perthes' disease was of multifactorial inheritance it would be expected that girls, being the more rarely affected, would have a higher proportion of affected relatives than boys. This is not found in Wynne-Davies' study.
4. It rarely involves the second twin.

Epidemiological factors

In a detailed study of cases by Wynne-Davies and Gormley (1978) a number of interesting facts have emerged.

1. There is no increased incidence of still birth or abortions in the families of these children.

2. Length of gestation and birth weight

Although low birth weight has been reported by Molloy and MacMahon (1967) and by Fisher (1972) in girls the incidence of true prematurity is the same as that in the general population. In a series of 25 premature babies there was only one case of bilateral disease. Thirty-two per cent had a family history of genito-urinary malformation, and in addition 28 per cent were delivered following breech presentation or had undergone version late in pregnancy for breech position. In the series as a whole an unexpected finding of 10 per cent breech presentation was present compared with 2–4 per cent for the normal population.

3. Parental age, parity and social class

The age of the parents of children with this condition is significantly higher than that found in the general population with fathers four years and mothers two years older than the expected norm. This was even more apparent in cases with bilateral disease. Similar observations have also been noted in scoliosis (Wynne-Davies 1975). There was a statistically significant increase of children born late in the families of low income (social classes 4 and 5). In the high income families the mothers were almost all over the age of thirty. Only one child in this group was of short stature.

Constitutional factors

1. Stature

A number of writers have noted that these children have abnormalities of height, weight, and skeletal maturation. Goff (1954) stated that some of these children were of short stature and had delayed bone age. Ralston (1955) confirmed these findings in a follow-up of 72 cases. Cameron and Izatt (1960) reported short stature but did not confirm the presence of delay in skeletal maturation. Weiner and O'Dell (1970) and Fisher (1972) noted that these children were of below average height for the mean population but that their weight was about or above the average. Molloy and MacMahon (1967) had found that many of these children were of low birth weight. In the study by Wynne-Davies and Gormley (1978) the index patients differed from normal controls with a significant number of children in the ten to fifty percentile group. An unexpected finding here was that during adolescence Wynne-Davies' population did not differ significantly from normal but when adult her index patients were again significantly smaller than the control population. Burwell et al (1978) had further pursued this problem demonstrating not only a loss of height in the index patients but also that the growth disturbance affects various parts of the body to a different extent. It is most exaggerated in the forearms, hands, tibiae and feet. By comparison the shoulders and pelvis are of normal size and the head comparatively large. On the basis of these observations, they postulate an intrauterine cause for this abnormality, and suggest that there is a growth disturbance in these children which becomes established possibly at the time of distal limb development. This theory is further supported by the fact that there is an increased incidence of associated congenital anomalies (Hall et al 1979).

2. *Skeletal age*

Although Goff (1954) was the first to describe growth abnormalities in this condition Girdany and Osman (1968) and Fisher (1972) were the first to comment in detail on the delayed skeletal maturation in these patients. Cavanagh et al (1936), however, had already noted delayed bone age but had attributed this fact to the presence of thyroid disorders. Harrison et al (1976) showed that the delay in skeletal age was present not only in the index patients but also in a number of their first degree relatives. With healing of the disease many of the patients returned to the normal bone age for chronological age but in others the delay in skeletal maturity persisted for a number of years after healing of the disease.

Associated anomalies

A number of authors (Fisher 1972, Wilk 1965, Catterall et al 1971 Matsoukas 1975, Wynne-Davies and Gormley 1978) have reported an association between congenital anomalies and Legg-Calvé-Perthes' disease. These vary from such major abnormalities as pyloric stenosis, congenital heart disease and epilepsy (Hall et al 1979, Wynne-Davies and Gormley 1978) and less serious abnormalities such as inguinal hernia and genito-urinary disease (Catterall et al 1971). Minor congenital anomalies have been fully reported by Hall et al (1979). They have shown that there is a significant difference in the incidence of these congenital anomalies in children with Legg-Calvé-Perthes' disease and normal controls. Many of these are related to socio-economic factors such as increased maternal age, family size and social status which may account for their presence in this condition.

1970 review

In 1970 I undertook a retrospective review of the notes and radiographs of 388 cases collected from many centres in the British Isles. Although this was undertaken primarily as a study of the radiological features the notes were carefully examined for a number of aetiological factors (Table 2.3). It is observed that there is an unexpectedly high incidence of both hernia, undescended testicle and genito-urinary disease in these patients. The expected incidence of inguinal hernia in the normal population is 7.9 per thousand (Knox 1959). These factors have already been reported (Catterall et al 1971) but this larger series confirms the findings. When the incidence of these abnormalities is examined within the radiological groups it is seen that their incidence varies. This tendency for renal anomalies is further exacerbated by summating Group I with Group IV and Group II with Group III (Table 2.4). Evidence will be presented

Table 2.3 Sex ratio and associated anomalies (1970 Survey)

	Total Number	No. of Boys	No. of Girls	Ratio of boys to girls	Renal anomalies	Hernia and undescended testicle
All cases	388	305	83	3.67:1	22	10
Unilateral cases	323	248	75	3.3 :1	12	8
Group I	30	28	2	14 :1	5	3
Group II	143	113	30	3.8 :1	2	3
Group III	107	75	32	2.3 :1	3	1
Group IV	43	32	11	2.9 :1	2	1
Bilateral cases	65	57	8	7 :1	10	2

Table 2.4 Incidence of renal tract and inguinal region abnormalities (1970 Survey)

	Groups I/IV	Groups II/III	Bilateral cases	Unilateral cases
Renal disease	+ 7	5	+ 10	12
	− 66	245	− 55	311
	$x^2 = 7.10^*$		$x^2 = 11.68^{**}$	
Hernia and undescended testicle	+ 4	4	+ 2	8
	− 56	184	− 55	240
	$x^2 + 1.72$ (N.S.)		$x^2 = 0.09$ (N.S.)	

$^*p = < 0.01$
$^{**}p = < 0.001$

in the Chapters on Morphology and Clinical features to support the view that Groups II and III are a spectrum of disease of common morphology and Groups I and IV may similarly represent another subtype. This latter type by contrast with Groups II and III appears to have a much higher incidence of associated abnormalities. Cases with bilateral involvement have a greater tendency for renal anomalies. In addition there is also a tendency for a greater proportion of these children to be born during the winter months although the explanation for this is not clear.

Conclusions

It is a conclusion of all these studies and reports that although the cause of this condition is not understood, there are both constitutional and environmental factors which collectively make the child more susceptible to this disease process.

Of the constitutional factors there are two features. There is the tendency in the patients and their relatives for an increased incidence of minor congenital anomalies, inguinal hernia and renal tract anomalies compared with normal controls. Secondly, there are growth disturbances. These are grossly observed as small stature and delayed bone age. A disturbance of normal growth, commencing before the onset of this disease, would be expected to be most obvious in those bones which were growing at the greatest rate at the time of its occurrence. It is known that the rate of bone growth varies. The tibia has reached half its final length by the age of six years (Lloyd-Roberts 1980) whereas the femur grows at a different rate (Stallard 1980). This concept could offer an alternative explanation for the observations made by Burwell et al (1978), where an intrauterine cause is postulated for the growth disturbance observed clinically. It will be seen when the pathology of this condition is discussed that there is evidence to suggest that there is an abnormality of ossification of cartilage during the repair process. Similar factors could be concerned in the mechanism of delay in bone age.

Of the environmental factors, firstly, there are children in low income families born of older parents and having a higher incidence of bilateral disease. Secondly, there are children born prematurely often by breach presentation, having a low incidence of bilateral disease. Renal disease appears more common in bilateral cases and is rare in girls.

REFERENCES

Barker D J P, Dixon E, Taylor J F 1978 Perthes' disease of the hip in three regions of England. Journal of Bone and Joint Surgery 60B: 478
Burwell R G, Dangerfield P H, Hall D J, Vernon C L, Harrison M H M 1978 Perthes' disease. An anthropometric study revealing impaired and disproportionate growth. Journal of Bone and Joint Surgery 60B: 461–477
Cameron J M Izatt M M 1960 Legg-Calvé-Perthes' disease. Scottish Medical Journal 5: 148–154
Catterall A 1970 Personal observations
Catterall A 1971 The natural history of Perthes' disease, Journal of Bone and Joint Surgery 53B: 37–53

Catterall A, Lloyd-Roberts G C, Wynne-Davies R 1971 Association of Perthes' disease with congenital anomalies of genito-urinary tract and inguinal region. Lancet i: 996–997

Cavanagh L A, Shelton E K, Sutherland R 1936 Metabolic studies in osteochondritis of the capital femoral epiphysis. Journal of Bone and Joint Surgery 18: 957

Edgren W 1965 Coxa plana. A clinical and radiological investigation with particular reference to the importance of the metaphyseal changes for the final shape of the proximal part of the femur. Acta Orthopaedica Scandinavica Suppl: 84

Fisher R L 1972 An epidemiological study of Legg-Perthes' disease. Journal of Bone and Joint Surgery 54A: 769–778

Girdany B R, Osman M Z 1968 Longitudinal growth and skeletal maturation in Perthes' disease. Radiol, Clin. North Am. 6: 245–251

Goff C W 1954 Legg-Calvé-Perthes' syndrome and related osteochondroses of youth. Charles C Thomas, Springfield, Illinois

Gray I M, Lowry B, Renwick D H G 1972 Incidence and genetics of Legg-Perthes' disease (Osteochondritis deformans) in British Columbia: evidence of polygenic determination. Journal of Medical Genetics 9: 197–202

Hall D J, Harrison M H M, Burwell R G 1979 Congenital abnormalities and Perthes' disease. Journal of Bone and Joint Surgery 61B: 18

Harper P S, Brotherton B J, Cochlin D 1976 Genetic risks in Perthes' disease. Clinical Genetics 10: 178–182

Harrison M H M, Turner M H, Jacobs P 1976 Skeletal immaturity in Perthes' disease. Journal of Bone and Joint Surgery 58B: 37–40

Helbo S 1953 Morbus Calvé-Perthes. Thesis, Copenhagen, Fyns Tidendes Bogtrykkeri, Odense

Knox G 1959 The incidence of inguinal hernia in Newcastle children. Archives of Disease of Childhood 34: 482–486

Lloyd-Roberts G C 1980 Personal communication

Matsoukas J A 1975 Viral antibody titres to Rubella in Coxa plana or Perthes' disease. Acta Orthopaedica Scandinavica 46: 957–962

Molloy M K, MacMahon B 1967 Birth weight and Legg-Perthes' disease. Journal of Bone and Joint Surgery 49A: 498–506

Phemister D B 1921 Operation for epiphysitis of the head of the femur (Perthes' disease). Findings and results. Archives of Surgery 2: 221–230

Ralston E L 1955 Legg-Perthes' disease and physical development. Journal of Bone and Joint Surgery 37A: 647

Stallard M 1980 Personal communication

Wansbrough R M, Carrie A W, Walker N F, Ruckerbauer G 1959 Coxa plana, its genetic aspects and results of treatment with the long Taylor walking caliper; a long-term follow-up study. Journal of Bone and Joint Surgery 41A: 135–146

Weiner D S, O'Dell H W 1970 Legg-Calvé-Perthes' disease. Observations on skeletal maturation. Clinical Orthopaedics and Related Research 68: 44–49

Wilk L H 1965 Juvenile osteochondrosis of the hip. Journal of the American Medical Association 192: 939–946

Wynne-Davies R 1975 Infantile idiopathic scoliosis. Causative factors, particularly in the first 6 months of life. Journal of Bone and Joint Surgery 57B: 138–141

Wynne-Davies R, Gormley J 1978 The aetiology of Perthes' disease. Journal of Bone and Joint Surgery 60B: 6–14

3

Morbid anatomy

Essential to many of the controversies that exist in this disease there is a fundamental lack of understanding of its basic pathology and morphology. Because of this, treatment must be based on a study of the radiological images and the imperfections of clinical judgement.

Historical review

Perthes (1913) considered that this disease was an osteochondritis, and emphasised that it was not tuberculous in nature. This view was supported by Schwarz (1914) and Edberg (1918). It remained for Phemister (1921) to report the presence of bone necrosis with intact overlying articular cartilage. He considered the condition was inflammatory in origin. This view was supported by the reports of Riedel (1922), Lang (1932), and Axhausen (1923). Phemister (1930) later described the repair of avascular bone by creeping replacement or substitution. Zemansky (1928) comprehensively reviewed all the available reported cases, and confirmed the presence of avascular bone, the intact overlying articular cartilage, and islands of cartilage within the epiphysis. He also considered that the changes were secondary to an infective process. Later authors, however, suggested that the bone necrosis was the result of mechanical interference with the blood supply and not infection. Opinion was divided as to whether this interference was with the arterial supply as the vessels approached the epiphysis on the side of the neck or obstruction to the venous drainage as suggested by Burrows (1941).

Jonaster (1953) reported biopsies taken during the course of the disease and confirmed the presence of an early bone necrosis with a subsequent repair process. These findings were confirmed by Larsen and Reiman (1973). Mizuno et al (1966) reported conclusions on large core biopsies of 40 cases of this condition. They concluded that in the initial stages 'there was a more or less extensive avascular necrosis in the capital nucleus without any tissue reaction'. In the intermediate and late stages there was an extensive repair process 'with profuse formation of fibrous tissues with an abundant revascularisation'. They comment in detail on the types of 'cartilagenous bone formation' within the femoral head during the repair process. McKibbin and Ralis (1974) reported the histological findings of the anterior part of the femoral head during the established phase of the disease. They concluded that the changes observed radiologically were the repair of an epiphyseal infarct. There was evidence to suggest that this infarct had occurred on at least two occasions. The concept of double infarction was also supported by biopsy material from Inoue and Ono (1976). Dolman and Bell (1973) reported a case in the early phases of the disease. Again their observations were confined to the anterior part of the femoral head. They confirmed the presence of bone necrosis and suggested that part of the increased radiological density in the epiphysis was due to bone dust in the necrotic marrow tissue. They did not discuss the aetiology of the necrosis. Jensen and Lauritzen (1976) reported two cases. In one there was evidence of two episodes of infarction, while in the other the histological appearances did not support this view. They discussed the possible mechanisms of ischaemia and concluded that a vascular disorder causing ischaemia of the femoral head did not explain all the clinical findings in Legg-Calvé-Perthes' disease.

There is considerable difference in the conclusions reached by these many reports and the reader is left confused as to whether the differences are those of interpretation or of an extremely variable pathology dependent on the part of the femoral head submitted to biopsy.

In an attempt to resolve these issues research has been directed to reproduce this disease experimentally. It has been known since the anatomical studies of Trueta (1957) and more recently those of Crock (1967) and Ogden (1974) that vessels reaching the epiphysis traverse the side of the femoral neck subperiosteally, later becoming incorporated into the bony substance of the neck with growth (Kemp 1980). Ligation of these vessels on the side of the femoral neck although inducing infarction of the epiphysis does not reproduce the variable nature of this disease (Freeman and England 19–9, Sanchis et al 1973). The results reported by Hennard et al (1970, 1971), Kemp (1973) and Singleton and Jones (1979) of ischaemia of the epiphysis of variable duration do present changes more comparable with those observed in the human condition. Catterall's classification (1971, 1981) of the radiological features and natural history of this condition suggest that the long-term prognosis is proportional to the degree of radiological involvement of the epiphysis. This suggests a variable process, a factor not previously considered in published reports.

It is the conclusion of this review that there are changes in both the articular cartilage and bony epiphysis which are a consequence of interference with their blood supply, but the mechanism of this interference is not clear. The ischaemia and infarction are followed by a process of repair which for the main part is responsible for the deformity of the femoral head.

The anatomy of the normal femoral head in the child and the consequence of infarction

Before considering the morphology of the active disease it is important to have a knowledge of the normal femoral head in the child and also the results of infarction induced experimentally in the femoral head of immature animals.

The anatomy of the normal epiphysis

The normal femoral head comprises a bony epiphysis with its overlying articular cartilage, the deep layers of which form a growing zone, together with an underlying growth plate and metaphysis. In the growing child the medial portion of the metaphysis lies within the femoral head and is covered by articular cartilage. On the lateral aspect very little of the upper metaphysis is included in the femoral head and therefore covered by articular cartilage (Fig. 3.1a).

In the infant there is a continuous growth plate from the medial side of the femoral head to the lateral edge of the trochanter (Fig. 3.2). By the age of 5 or 6 years, there is a well-formed femoral neck with a growth plate over its proximal end and overlapping its lateral corner for a few millimetres only.

Morphologically the articular cartilage is composed of a superficial and deep zone. The deep zone or growing area (Fig. 3.1c) is capable of proliferation and is responsible for the overall enlargement of the femoral head during growth. It is ossified by an endochondral front from its deep surface. This bone is later remodelled to form trabecular bone. The superficial zone is responsible for the process of movement and lubrication only.

The bony trabeculae (Fig. 3.1b) within the epiphysis are thin and in the resting state do not show evidence of remodelling. They radiate out to the surface of the subchondral bone plate from the centre of the superior margin of the growth plate in its midpoint. Trabeculae lateral to this point appear to run horizontally at the level of the growth plate and to be somewhat thickened. A process of endochondral ossification is observed from the superior border of the growth plate in children up to the age of 5 years. This produces loss of vertical height of the growth plate seen in radiographs of the femoral head between the ages of 1 and 5 years.

Blood supply to the proximal femoral epiphysis

With the establishment of a bony epiphysis within the cartilagenous analogue of the femoral head the blood supply of this region becomes altered with

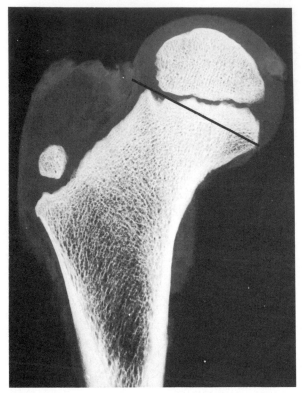

Fig. 3.1(a) Fine detail radiograph of mid-coronal section of the femoral head of a child aged 6 years. The line marks the lower margin of the femoral head. The medial side of the metaphysis lies within the femoral head.

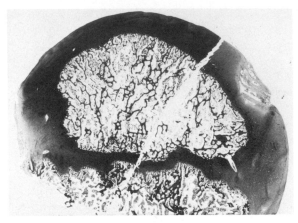

Fig. 3.1(b) Low power view × 2 of transverse section of femoral head of the same child stained with haemotoxylin and eosin. The thickened articular cartilage on the inferomedial aspect of the femoral head covers the medial metaphysis.

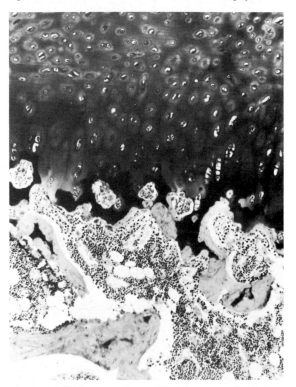

Fig. 3.1(c) High power view × 56 of deep zone of articular cartilage showing the growing zone and the endochondral ossification.

the formation of medial and lateral retinacular systems arising from the medial and lateral circumflex femoral arteries. The reader is referred to the excellent papers by Trueta (1957) and more recently Crock (1967) and Ogden (1974) for a detailed description of these vessels. Ogden (1974) has shown that between the ages of 3 and 8 years the major blood supply to the upper femoral epiphysis is via superior and inferior retinacular vessels arising from the medial circumflex femoral artery (Fig. 3.3). The lateral circumflex femoral supplies the greater trochanteric area, the anterior aspect of the neck and a very small portion of the anterior aspect of the epiphysis (Fig. 3.3). These vessels transverse the neck subperiosteally and later become incorporated within the bony substance of the femoral neck with growth (Kemp 1980). Interference with these vessels could occur at three possible sites; firstly, from the medial circumflex femoral shortly after it has left the profunda artery; secondly, to the medial circumflex femoral as it passes on the inferior aspect of the femoral neck when it can be compressed against the capsule by the psoas and finally on the femoral

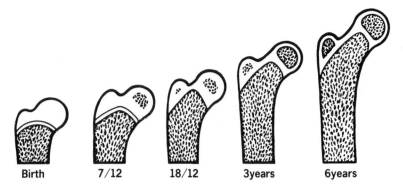

Fig. 3.2 Drawing of the growth of the upper end of the femur in the normal child.

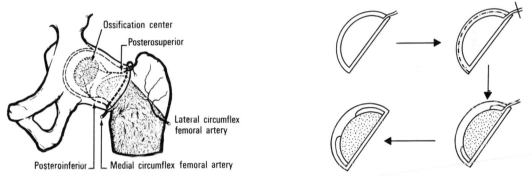

Fig. 3.3 Drawing of blood supply to the upper portion of the femur (After J.A. Ogden 1974).

Fig. 3.4 Drawing of the changes occurring in the upper femoral epiphysis after interference with the blood supply.

neck itself, either as the result of tamponade due to effusion or as a consequence of capsular compression by the position of abduction and internal rotation. Once the vessels have become incorporated in the substance of the femoral neck compression in this area would not occur.

The consequences of infarction of the upper femoral epiphysis

Infarction of the upper femoral epiphysis can be experimentally produced by interference with the retinacular system of vessels before they enter the epiphysis, either by a ligature placed around the femoral neck (Freeman 1969), or by tamponade compressing these vessels in the same region (Hennard 1970, 1971, Kemp 1973, Singleton and Jones 1979).

As the result of this ischaemia the bony epiphysis becomes necrotic and the marrow also dies. This results in cessation of the normal growth.

Although the bony epiphysis dies the overlying articular cartilage, being nourished by synovial fluid, continues to proliferate. This results in thickening of the cartilage (Fig. 3.4). This thickening occurs to a greater extent on the medial and lateral aspects of the femoral head than over the dome of the femoral head (Gershuni-Gordon and Axer 1974). Because of the increased thickness small areas of cartilage necrosis are seen in the deepest layers of the articular cartilage. This is due to the distance that the nutrients traverse through the articular cartilage to reach these cells.

Once the blood supply to the femoral epiphysis is re-established an invading vascular granulation tissue replaces the epiphyseal marrow. This granulation tissue resorbs part of the bony trabeculae after which apositional new bone formation produces trabecular thickening seen radiologically as an increase in density of the epiphysis (Bobechko and Harris 1968; Fig. 3.4). This process is called 'Creeping replacement or substitution' (Phemister

1930). In the thickened overlying articular cartilage the process of endochondral ossification is seen starting in the region of the perichondrial ring tissue and spreading upwards over the epiphysis (Fig. 3.4). A vertical section taken through the epiphysis at this time will show three appearances. Firstly, centrally and superiorly there are necrotic trabeculae surrounded by marrow which has not been revascularised; secondly, there is in the deeper part of the epiphysis the process of creeping substitution with a vascular tissue replacing the marrow and new bone formation laid on the framework of the vascular trabeculae; thirdly, in the periphery of the femoral head there is viable trabecular bone which does not show evidence of avascular necrosis but may show remodelling.

REVIEW OF HUMAN CASE MATERIAL

Bearing in mind the very varied radiological appearances of this process and the thought that the prognosis is proportional to the degree of radiological involvement (Ch. 5), I resolved that a better understanding of the human morphological appearances would be gained by a review of as much human material as possible. I was, indeed, fortunate through the generosity of the authors of previously published cases to obtain a total of four femoral heads and five core biopsies. In one case the opposite uninvolved hip was available for comparison. In addition, five normal heads were obtained to act as normal controls (Table 3.1).

The uninvolved hip

Although only one involved hip is available for study, when this is compared with a normal control of comparable age a number of interesting observations were obtained.

1. Articular cartilage. When compared with normal controls the articular cartilage was of increased thickness and showed small islands of calcification throughout its substance. The growing zone on the deep surface was macroscopically present and did not differ significantly from the histological appearance of the normal control (Figs. 3.5a and b).

2. The growth plate. Although in general the

Table 3.1

Case	Source	Group	Stage		
Whole femoral heads					
A	Mckibbin	II	Active	Anterior half of femoral head	J.B.J.S. 56B: 438–447
B	Lloyd-Roberts	III	Healing	Whole femoral head	Unpublished
C	Dolman and Bell	III	Active	Anterior half Posterior half	J.B.J.S. 55A: 184–188 Unpublished
D	Fulford	III	Healing	Whole head	Unpublished
Core biopsies					
E	Kemp	IV	Active	Femoral head and neck	Unpublished
F	Kemp	IV	Active	Femoral head and neck	Unpublished
G	Ponseti	III	Active	Femoral head and neck	J.B.J.S. 38A: 739–750
H	Ponseti	IV	Active	Femoral head and neck	J.B.J.S. 38A: 739–750
I	Ponseti	III	Active	Femoral head and neck	Unpublished
Opposite normal hips					
J	Fulford	—	—	Whole femoral head	Unpublished

Normal control
5 Normal femoral heads between 4 and 9 years.

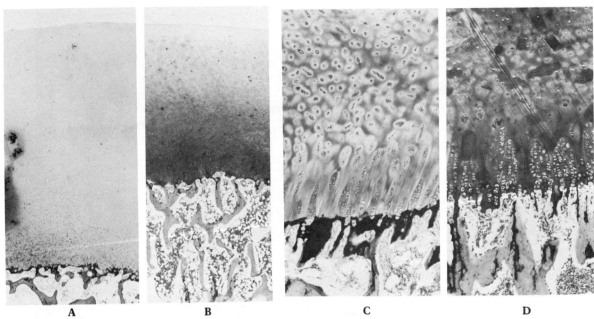

Fig. 3.5 Case D — uninvolved hip. (a) Low power view × 11 of articular cartilage. Areas of calcification are seen in the substance of the cartilage. The difference in thickness compared with normal controls (b) is noted. (b) Low power view × 11 of articular cartilage from normal control hip of child of similar age.

Fig. 3.5(c) Case D — uninvolved hip. High power view × 42 of growth plate. There is some distortion of the cell columns. It is observed that in some regions the cell columns are absent. The endochondral ossification on the metaphyseal side of these areas is abnormal. (d) High power view × 42 of normal growth plate.

microscopical appearance of the growth plate was normal there were areas where there was considerable distortion of the normal anatomy suggesting a minor degree of mechanical deformation of the plate. The ossification on its deep surface was proceeding normally but there was more unossified cartilage in the primary trabeculae than is seen in normal controls (Fig. 3.5c and d).

3. *The bony epiphysis.* The anatomical arrangements in the trabeculae were similar to that in the normal control. The marrow showed some slight fatty replacement but haemopoetic tissue was also seen.

This case suggests that in the uninvolved hip in this condition there are histological abnormalities to be observed. There is thickening of the articular cartilage and some distortion of the architecture of the growth plate. These findings would suggest that this femoral head may be predisposed to disease. Thickened articular cartilage has been shown by Greshuni-Gordon and Axer (1974) to be associated with deformity of the femoral head without an abnormality of the bony epiphysis itself. It is interesting to observe that in

a number of other sites there is delayed ossification as instanced by a delay in bone age seen particularly in the hands and the feet.

Involved femoral heads

Each case was grouped to assess the extent of radiological involvement and also staged to decide whether the disease was in the active or healing phase (Table 3.1). There were no early cases available showing the subchondral fracture line. In the case reported by Dolman and Bell death had occurred within a few months of the onset of symptoms. These were the earliest changes observed in the Groups II and III cases. No Group I case was available for study, the morphological appearances of the remaining Groups will be discussed according to the degree of radiological involvement.

Groups II/III

These two Groups will be considered together as they represent a common morphological process in

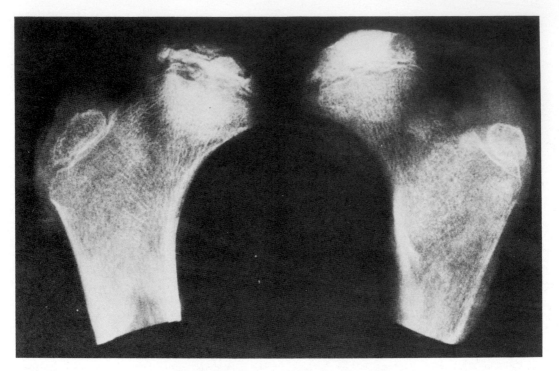

Fig. 3.6 Case C — Dolman and Bell. Radiographs of the anterior and posterior halves of the femoral head. There is considerable flattening of the bony epiphysis in the anterior half, while in the posterior half of the head there is a central area of density with collapse with more normally textured bone on the medial and lateral aspects. (Produced by permission of the Board of Trustees of the Journal of Bone and Joint Surgery.)

the early stages. There is only one example of early disease in this Group which is the case reported by Dolman and Bell. The radiographs (Fig. 3.6) of this case show typical early Group III appearances with loss of epiphyseal height but an apparent preservation of normally textured bone on the medial, lateral and posterior aspects of the epiphysis. There is sclerosis in the central and anterior areas of the epiphysis suggesting crushing of the bony trabeculae. Histologically in the anterior part of the femoral head the overlying articular cartilage is thickened and the bony epiphysis appears to be completely crushed with large numbers of necrotic and fractured trabeculae. The necrotic marrow tissue appears calcified or full of bone dust. There are very small areas of intact but necrotic bone immediately overlying the growth epiphysis. In the posterior part of the femoral head an entirely different appearance is seen (Fig. 3.7a). The overlying articular cartilage is thickened but this is particularly apparent on the medial and the lateral aspects of the femoral head. Under high power the articular cartilage shows areas of calcification similar to that seen in the uninvolved hip. In the bony epiphysis a number of distinct areas are observed.

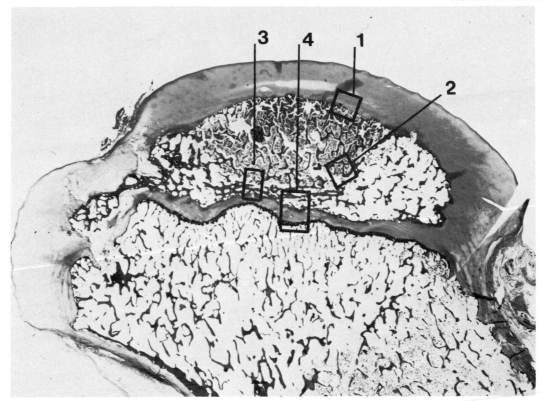

Fig. 3.7(a) Low power view × 7 of a coronal section taken from the posterior part of the femoral head of Case D stained with haemotoxylin and eosin. The articular cartilage is thickened, particularly on the medial and lateral aspects of the femoral head. The defect on the medial side is for the attachment of the ligamentum tares and the configuration of the bony trabeculae in this area is normal for this portion of the femoral head. The dense central area is composed partly of crushed trabeculae and partly of necrotic marrow which is itself showing evidence of calcification.

1. On the medial and lateral aspects of the epiphysis the trabeculae, although a little thickened and showing evidence of remodelling, are intact and show no evidence of necrotic bone.

2. In the central area of the epiphysis the bony trabeculae appear thickened, crushed and necrotic. This necrotic marrow is radiologically dense suggesting that it is calcified. The overlying articular cartilage is viable but the growing zone on the deep surface is in areas necrotic (Fig. 3.7b). A few of the deep cells of the articular cartilage are also necrotic.

3. The junctional zone between the necrotic tissue and the viable areas show a vascular granulation tissue invading into the necrotic and crushed bone. In areas where the trabecular structure is intact apositional new bone formation is being laid on the framework of a vascular trabeculae. (Fig. 3.7c).

4. In the area deep to the crushed zone and above the growth plate, horizontally running trabeculae, thickened and many showing evidence of avascular necrosis with apositional new bone formation, are seen (Fig. 3.7d).

The growth plate is abnormal. There is loss of

B

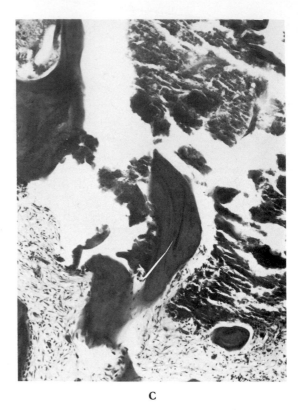

C

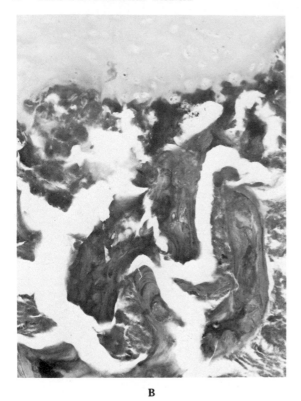

D

Fig. 3.7(b) High power view × 63 of area stained with haemotoxylin and eosin. This shows the thickened necrotic trabeculae with necrotic marrow on the deep surface of the articular cartilage. The normal growing zone has been lost.

Fig. 3.7(c) High power view × 63 of area 2 stained with haemotoxylin and eosin. This shows the revascularisation front invading the infarcted zone. There is appositional bone on the surface of the trabeculae that are already revascularised.

Fig. 3.7(d) High power view × 63 of area 3 stained with haemotoxylin and eosin. This region just above the growth plate shows thickened horizontally running trabeculae showing central necrosis with appositional new bone which is viable. The marrow is revascularised.

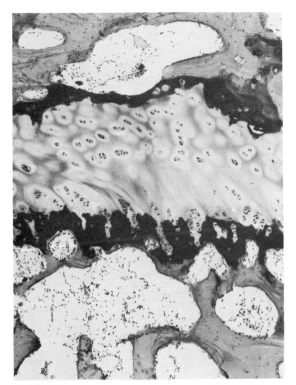

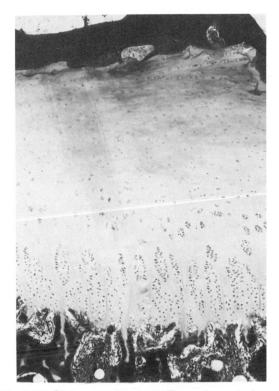

Fig. 3.8(a) High power view × 50 of the growth plate in area 4 stained with haemotoxylin and eosin. There is loss of the normal resting zone of the growth plate and distortion of the columns which are also shorter than normal. The overlying trabeculae in this area do show evidence of remodelling but not of avascular necrosis.

Fig. 3.8(b) High power view × 50 of normal growth plate stained with haemotoxylin and eosin.

its height and distortion of the normal contour of the cell columns. There is no penetration of the growth plate by vascular channels (Fig. 3.8a and b).

When the appearances seen histologically are considered three dimensionally we find that the viable bone is situated on the medial, lateral and posterior aspects of the head with the zone of infarc-

tion lying in the centre. The necrotic trabeculae are situated along the growth plate anteriorly and rising posteriorly to blend the viable trabeculae. The zone of crushed necrotic trabeculae is in direct relation to this and thicker anteriorly than it is posteriorly. (Fig. 3.9).

These appearances are those of incomplete infarct with continuing growth of those portions of

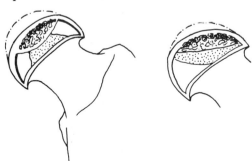

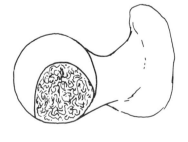

Fig. 3.9 Drawing of the morphological appearances in Groups II and III cases. The clear area represents viable trabeculae which show remodelling only. The stippled shading represents trabeculae with central necrosis and appositional new bone. The irregular shading corresponds to the area of crushed necrotic trabeculae.

the epiphysis which remain viable. This infarction is followed by a process of repair and remodelling. This may be complicated by further episodes of infarction caused by mechanical interference of the blood supply in areas of trabecular fracture. Because the ischaemia interferes with the normal ossification of the deep zone of the articular cartilage, persisting growth of this tissue which is nourished by synovial fluid will result in an increase in its thickness. This thickened cartilage being biologically plastic is moulded by position and movement. With collapse of the bony epiphysis, particularly in its anterior part, deformity of the femoral head will occur.

Healing phases

As the disease progresses the changes observed are proportional to three factors: the extent of the infarcted bone and therefore the size of bone remaining viable; the extent of the crushing of the necrotic bone; and the overgrowth of the articular cartilage occurring as a consequence of the initial episode of infarction. These factors may be compared and contrasted by consideration of cases B and D which represent the histological appearances occurring during healing of the disease without femoral head deformity (Figs. 3.10 and 3.11).

Following infarction of the bony epiphysis a repair process becomes apparent which, in the main part, is confined to the area of necrotic bone. The trabecular tissues which remain intact are invaded by a vascular granulation tissue which initially resorbs part of the trabeculae and then lays appositional new bone on its surface, a process termed 'Creeping Substitution' (Phemister 1930) (Fig.

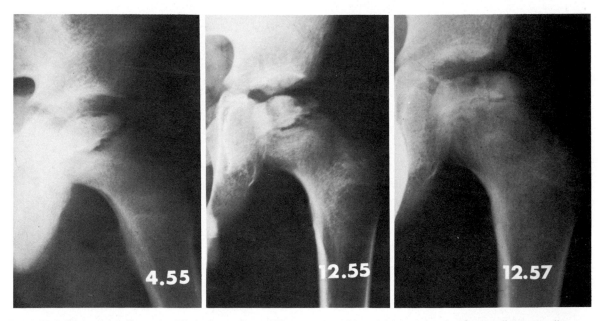

Fig. 3.10(a) The serial radiographs. These show a Group III appearance with an initial subchondral fracture line proceeding to an extensive area of reabsorption with large viable medial and small lateral fragments. In the radiographs, December 1957, healing was well established.

Fig. 3.10 Case B history: child aged 10 years when Legg-Calvé-Perthes' disease of the left hip was diagnosed incidentally during the investigation of renal tract anomalies. Routine urine examination revealed a heavy protinuria and nephrotic syndrome was subsequently diagnosed due to underlying chronic nephritis. Despite conservative therapy by a low salt diet his renal state deteriorated. He died of uraemia and hypertension at the age of 12 years 6 months. His Legg-Calvé-Perthes' disease had been treated by a weight-relieving caliper for a period of 6 months only. At necropsy the changes of chronic glomerular nephritis, hypertension, uraemia, pericarditis and pleurisy were found. Macroscopically the femoral head showed some distortion with flattening of the superior and lateral margin of the head. The cartilage in this area appeared fibrillated.

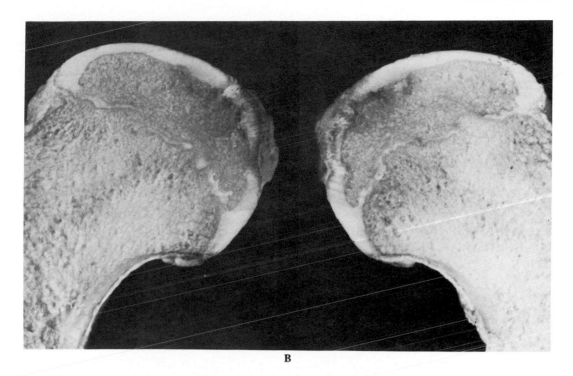

B

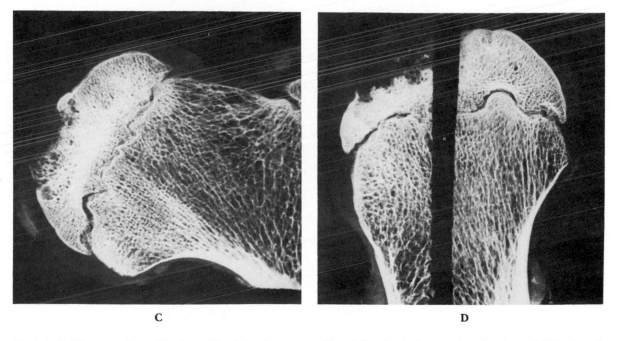

C

D

Fig. 3.10(b) The cut surfaces of the femoral head showing an area of fatty infiltration in the metaphyseal region and thickening of the articular cartilage, particularly on the medial and lateral side.

Fig. 3.10(c) Slab radiograph of mid-coronal section of the femoral head and neck.

Fig. 3.10(d) Slab radiographs of anterior and posterior slabs cut at right angles to coronal plane, the gap between them represents the portion of the femoral head removed for slabs.

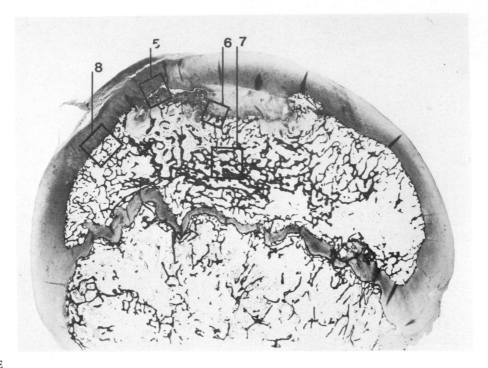

E

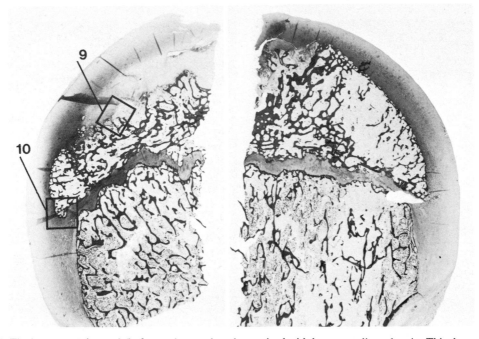

F

Fig. 3.10(e) The low power view × 2.5 of central coronal section, stained with haemotoxylin and eosin. This shows thickening of the articular cartilage. The trabeculae on the medial and lateral aspects of the epiphysis appear normal. The trabeculae in the central area above the growth plate are thickened and there is a defect in the superior part of the head which appears to be fibrocartilagenous in nature and to have fissures within it.

Fig. 3.10(f) Low power view × 2.5 of the anterior and posterior parts of the femoral head corresponding to the slab radiograph. In the posterior part of the head the trabeculae appear normal, the thickened zone appears to be wedge-shaped, spreading forward along the line of the growth plate. The defect seen on the superior part of the coronal section is an extensive area of fibrocartilage reaching well forward into the anterior part of the epiphysis. It is being ossified from its deep surface. There is an area of endochondral ossification in the anterior part of the thickened articular cartilage.

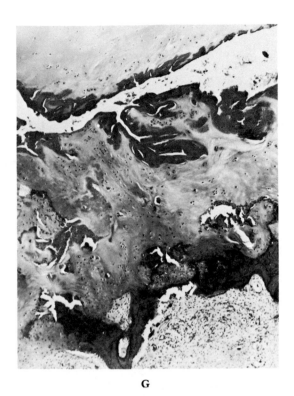

G

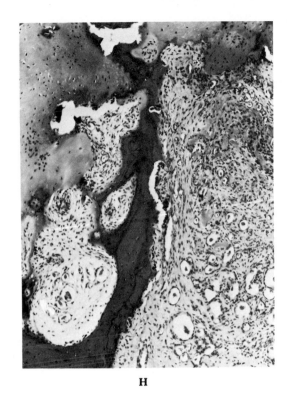

H

Fig. 3.10(g) High power view × 75 of area 5. The fissure defect in the articular cartilage is noted. The cartilagenous material deep to this is being eroded by vascular granulation tissue.

Fig. 3.10(h) High power view × 75 of area 6. This shows the fibrocartilagenous material being actively invaded by granulation tissue in which a number of giant cells can be seen, the appearances are consistent with changes seen in hyperparathyroidism.

Fig. 3.10(i) High power view × 60 of area 7. The thickened trabeculae show extensive evidence of remodelling but no evidence of osteocyte death.

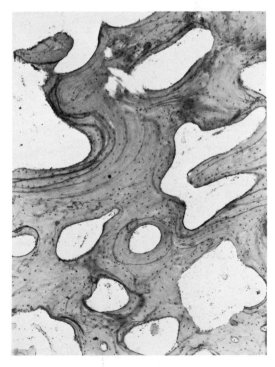

I

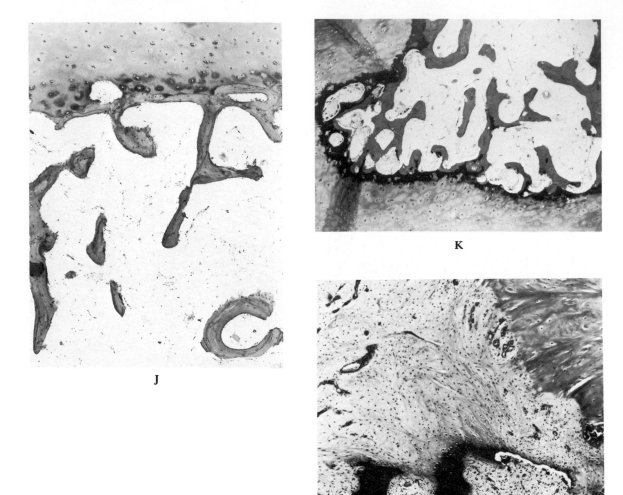

J

K

L

Fig. 3.10(j) High power view × 60 of area 8 shows that the growing zone on the deep surface of the articular cartilage and the subchondral are normal. The trabeculae showing some evidence of remodelling. There is no evidence of hyperparathyroid changes in these sections.

Fig. 3.10(k) High power view × 52 of area 9. On the right side of the section is the fibrocartilagenous material which is being eroded by a vascular granulation tissue behind which woven bone is forming. There are some giant cells to be seen.

Fig. 3.10(l) High power view × 52 of area 10 showing a typical endochondral ossification front occurring in the thickened articular cartilage of the anterior part of the femoral head.

When the sequential radiographs, the slab radiographs and the histological appearances are compared it would seem that the normally textured trabeculae on the medial, posterior and lateral aspects of the femoral head have been present throughout the disease process but continuing to enlarge by normal growth. The area of fibrocartilagenous material corresponds approximately to the area of necrotic crushed bone in the epiphysis. The almost complete absence of necrotic bone in the central area could be due to simple remodelling as bone turnover in this area appears rapid, but peripherally the bone appears neither thick nor seriously remodelled. These findings suggest that only part of the epiphysis was actually infarcted, the remainder remaining viable. The area of remodelling is confined to those trabeculae which have probably been avascular but not crushed. Those trabeculae which have been crushed have been removed and replaced by fibrocartilagenous material.

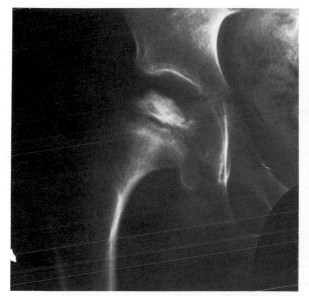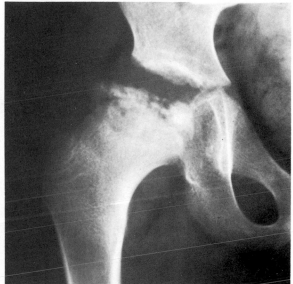

A

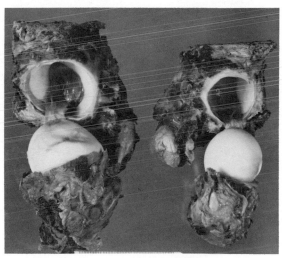

B

Fig. 3.11 Case D history. A child aged 8 years who developed a painful right-sided limp and subsequent investigation revealed Legg-Calvé-Perthes' disease: Group III. Routine investigation showed a raised E.S.R. and subsequently lymphocytic lymphoma was diagnosed. The lymphoma was treated by chemotherapy, but the hip remained untreated and serial radiographs showed progressive head deformity. Despite adequate chemotherapy his lymphoma later relapsed and he died of bronchopneumonia. At this time the Legg-Calvé-Perthes' disease was in the healing phase.

Fig. 3.11(a) The serial radiographs taken at the time of diagnosis and shortly before death, 18 months later, show a Group III appearance with a large involved segment but small normally textured medial fragment. The final radiographs show that the condition was in the healing phase with almost complete reabsorption of the dense central fragment.

Fig. 3.11(b) The excised hip joints. There is a considerable degree of deformity of both the femoral head and acetabulum on the involved side. There is a striking enlargement of the femoral head on the involved side and a dent on its anterior and lateral aspect.

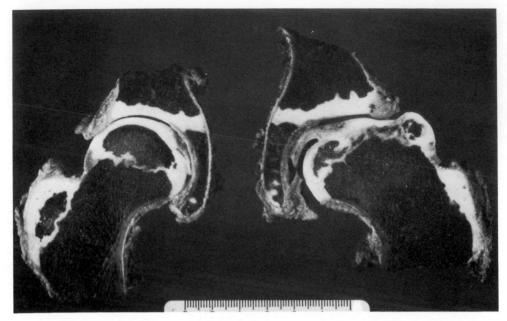

C

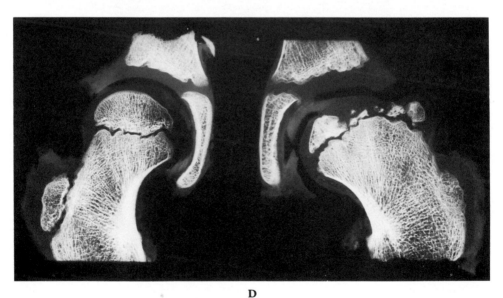

D

Fig. 3.11(c) Photographs of 0.5 cm slabs taken from the centre of the femoral head and acetabulum. On the involved side the femoral head deformity is observed and the point of impingement of the lateral acetabular lip on the femoral head. On the uninvolved side the cartilage on the medial and lateral aspects of the femoral head appears thick compared with normal controls.

Fig. 3.11(d) Radiograph of the above specimen.

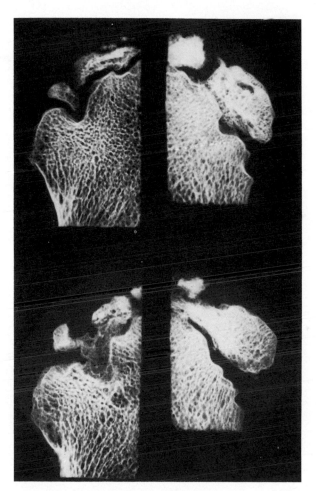

Fig. 3.11(e) Radiographs of slabs taken in the sagittal plane of the anterior and posterior parts of the femoral head. The upper pair are from the lateral aspect of the head and the lower pair from the medial side of the femoral head.

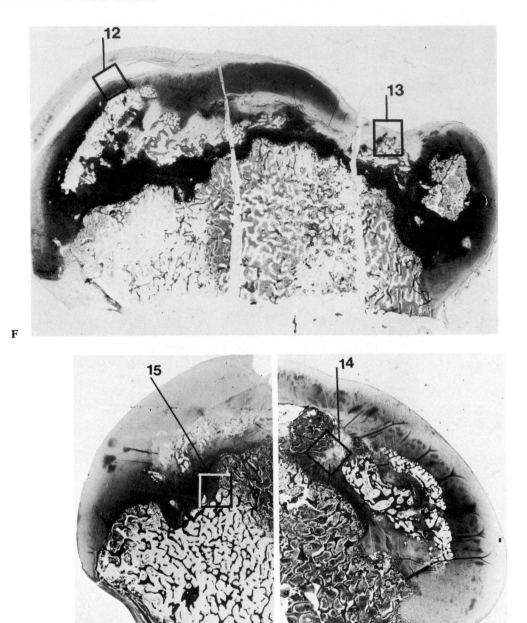

Fig. 3.11(f) Low power view × 2.5 of the transverse section of the femoral head. The deformity of the femoral head is noted with a complete loss of the articular cartilage in the region of the dent. On the medial and lateral sides of the femoral head there is endochondral new bone formation in the thickened articular cartilage. The bone in the central area of the epiphysis is thickened but does not show evidence of avascular necrosis but does show remodelling. There is a large quantity of fibrocartilagenous material deep to the articular cartilage in the centre of the epiphysis.

Fig. 3.11(g) Low power view × 3.5 of the anterior and posterior parts of the femoral head. In the anterior half a large metaphyseal lesion can be seen. In the posterior section there is an area of necrotic and crushed bone, with calcification of the necrotic marrow. This area is dense on the fine detail radiograph. In the posterior aspect of the section there is a superficial area of endochondral new bone formed in the thickened articular cartilage. Deep to this is an area of thickened trabecular bone showing remodelling but no evidence of avascular necrosis.

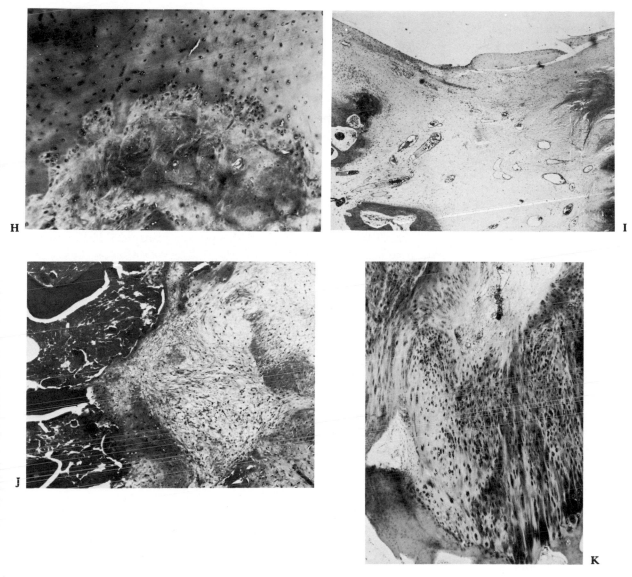

Fig. 3.11(h) High power view × 34 of area 12. This shows the articular cartilage has been remodelled from its deep surface by a fibrocartilagenous material.

Fig. 3.11(i) High power view × 20 of area 13. This shows the region of the dent in the femoral head showing a complete loss of the normal articular cartilage with fibrillation of the surface. There is a layer of cells covering the surface of the fibrocartilage reminiscent of Pannus.

Fig. 3.11(j) High power view × 45.5 of area 14. This shows the granulation tissue invading the necrotic marrow and trabecular bone. Giant cells are visible. Fibrocartilage appears to be forming in the areas behind the zone of reabsorption.

Fig. 3.11(k) High power view × 30 of area 15. This shows the lower margin of the metaphyseal lesion with gross distortion of the architecture of the growth plate and almost complete absence of the normal endochondral ossification expected in this area.

As in Case E the conclusion may be reached that there is an area of trabecular bone in the posterior and medial aspect of the epiphysis which shows evidence of remodelling without definite avascular necrosis. The femoral head has been deformed mainly in an anterior and lateral direction and new bone has formed by endochondral ossification in the thickened deformed articular cartilage. This is well formed laterally as a mass of trabecular bone passing postero-medially as a thin tongue in the thickened articular cartilage and overlying the viable posterior medial trabecular bone of the original epiphysis. These appearances are consistent with an incomplete infarct but of much greater extent than in the previous case.

3.7d). In those areas where the trabeculae become crushed and in which mechanical deformation is also occurring, the vascular granulation tissue is unable to invade the infarcted zone. These necrotic trabeculae are therefore reabsorbed from their deep surface by giant-cell osteoclasts (Fig. 3.11j). The fibrous tissue so formed is converted into a fibrocartilagenous material which appears to be able to proliferate under load and is biologically plastic, adapting its shape to that of the acetabulum in which it lies. This repair process, therefore, is different from that of creeping substitution and deposits a fibrocartilagenous material in those areas where the trabeculae are necrotic and crushed; a process thought of as 'Chondrification of the Infarct'. There is in these circumstances a progressive loss of height in the epiphysis as the necrotic bone is removed. This accounts for the continuing collapse observed radiologically during the active phase of the disease. These findings are best observed in Case B reported by Ralis and McKibbin.

The articular cartilage being nourished by synovial fluid continues to proliferate and this will result in an increased thickness of the cartilage, the degree of which seems to be proportional to the degree of ischaemia. Possibly due to biomechanical causes this thickening of the articular cartilage occurs mainly on the medial and the lateral aspects of the femoral head, and on the lateral side this reactivates the growth plate on the lateral aspect of the femoral neck present in the younger child. The effect of this proliferation and moulding produces overgrowth of the femoral head laterally, reported radiologically as subluxation.

Group IV

In this Group only core biopsies are available for study — Cases E, F, H. They all, however, show a similar appearance and are in the active phases of the disease. The radiographs show that there is considerable flattening of the bony epiphysis with some loss of height in distance between the growth plate and the roof of the acetabulum. This suggests femoral head deformity. Histologically the core biopsy shows thickening of the articular cartilage, the cells of which are largely viable, although there are occasional cells in the deep

zone which are necrotic. The bony trabeculae are crushed and necrotic immediately deep to the articular cartilage. Below this they are also necrotic but show gross thickening with several cement lines (Fig. 3.12). The crushing may be the result of the technique of biopsy by trephine but as the radiological features suggest crushing of the bony epiphysis the appearances almost certainly antidate the biopsy. The marrow also appears infarcted and there is no evidence of an invading granulation tissue in the material obtained. The growth plate also shows abnormalities. The resting zone is extremely thin. On the metaphyseal side, there are columns of cartilagenous cells streaming down from the growth plate unossified into the metaphyseal region. This may offer an explanation for the wide growth plate seen in these cases.

The thickened necrotic trabeculae, with evidence of remodelling as instanced by numerous cement lines, suggest recurrent episodes of total ischaemia of the epiphysis. This would suggest a rather more complete ischaemia of the epiphysis than that seen in the Groups II/III cases and that the ischaemia might even be of a recurrent nature.

Two possible mechanisms could account for the radiological appearances seen in this Group (Fig. 3.13). In the younger child total infarction of the bony epiphysis with overgrowth of the articular cartilage would give a small epiphysis with a normal space between the growth plate and acetabulum (E.A) (Catterall 1971). As the blood supply is re-established ossification would occur lateral to the epiphysis in this thickened articular cartilage. This repair phase could again be complicated by further episodes of infarction. In the older child a bony epiphysis of greater size might be subject to total collapse following infarction of the epiphysis and the loose trabeculae then removed, giving a similar appearance in the long term.

Metaphyseal changes

Ponseti (1956) is the only author to comment in detail on the nature of metaphyseal lesions. Very little has been written in the past on these metaphyseal changes and it was felt to be particularly important to make observations on these lesions. There were various common factors in the cases observed.

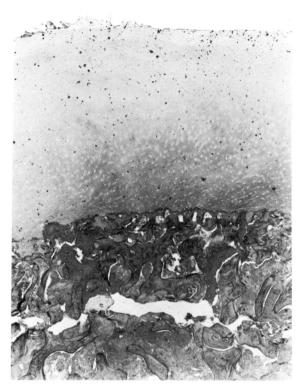

Fig. 3.12(a) Case E. Group IV. Low power view × 17.5. There is thickening of the bony trabeculae which are also crushed. Both the marrow and the bone are necrotic.

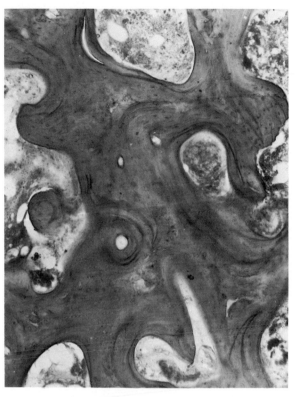

Fig. 3.12(b) High power view × 61 of thickened trabeculae. There are several cement lines suggesting remodelling but complete necrosis of the bone and the marrow.

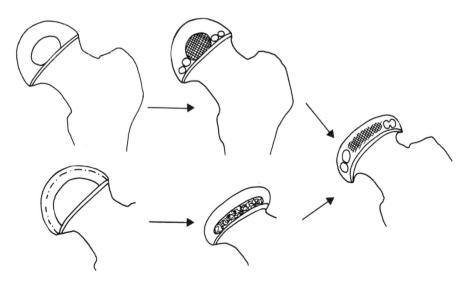

Fig. 3.13 Drawing of the possible mechanisms producing a change in head shape in the Group IV cases in the younger and older child.

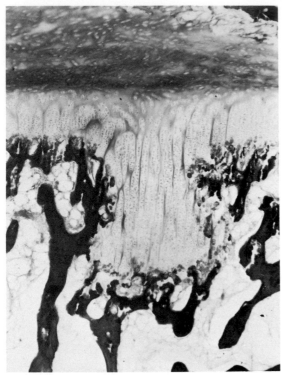

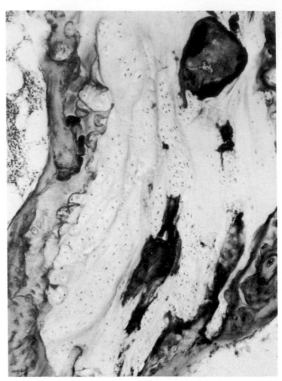

Fig. 3.14 Case B. Low power view × 25.5 of a localised metaphyseal lesion. The thinning of the growth plate is observed and columns of cells passing down into the metaphyseal region unossified are noted. Thick trabecular bone surrounds this lesion.

Fig. 3.15 A high power view × 96 of the edge of a metaphyseal lesion showing proliferation of the cartilagenous cells and the thickened surrounding bone.

1. In all cases in which the disease process was active there was an area of fatty replacement of the marrow situated in the central part of the metaphyseal region. This area may correspond approximately to the shape of the metaphysis at the onset of the disease. In this area the normal marrow cells were replaced by fat and there were more osteoid seams visible in the trabeculae by comparison with the normal controls. There were occasional areas of cellular infiltration with plasma cells and lymphocytes. The trabeculae showed no serious evidence of remodelling.

2. In Cases D, G, H, and I the radiographs showed a circumscribed lesion with a well-defined sclerotic margin. These lesions are only seen during the active phase of the disease. Histologically, the appearances were those of a fibrocartilagenous material with a surrounding area of reactive new bone formation. The material morphologically is very similar to that seen in the reabsorbed area of the epiphysis. This lesion appears to be an active lesion with cells capable of proliferation (Fig. 3.15).

3. In Case H radiologically the growth plate appeared to be wide in places with no clear cut deep border with the metaphysis. Histologically, this area shows disorganised endochondral ossification without evidence of ischaemia on the metaphyseal side of the plate. The cartilage columns were observed streaming unossified into the metaphysis. This process seems to be failure of normal endochondral ossification without evidence of interference with the blood supply. Where a localised metaphyseal lesion is in direct contact with the growth plate the whole architecture of the plate is lost and there is no ossification on its deep surface (Fig. 3.12k). This will lead to different rates of growth of the femoral neck and hence contribute to femoral head deformity.

4. By contrast in the case reported by Jensen and Lauritzen (1976) there was one area on the medial side of the metaphysis in which there was

evidence of avascular necrosis with remodelling. The periosteal tissue in this area was a thrombosed retinacular vessel which they considered to be related to this process. This is the only case reported showing this change.

5. Finally in cases showing femoral head deformity on the lateral side of the metaphysis the lateral part of the enlarged cartilagenous portion of the femoral head covers the metaphysis. On its deep surface is a normal growth plate. This will induce lateral growth of the neck and further enlargement of the femoral head. In Case D, at the angle between this area and the original growth plate it is breached by bone. This bony bridge is an area of premature growth arrest and the presence of this change will produce further deformity of the femoral head.

Discussion of human case material

Two aspects of this material merit further discussion at this stage. These are the extent of the infarction within the epiphysis and the process of repair.

This evidence suggests that the ischaemic process produces a variable degree of infarction of the epiphyseal bone. In Groups II and III the volume of bone remaining viable is too great to have been formed by endochondral ossification in thickened articular cartilage and radiologically appears to be part of the original epiphysis. Incomplete infarction of the femoral head is a well-established pattern of pathology in the adult forms of avascular necrosis of the femoral head (Catto 1976, Inoue and Ono 1979).

Henard (1970, 1971) has reproduced in dogs changes very similar to those seen in the present series of cases by periods of ischaemia of 6, 8 and 10 hours duration. In particular, the changes following 8 hours of ischaemia are of interest. The trabeculae in the central area of the epiphysis become avascular and are invaded by a vascular connective tissue which replaces the marrow and removes the central avascular trabeculae. However, in the subchondral area and in the trabeculae next to the growth plate there is appositional new bone producing thickening of the trabeculae. The bony epiphysis surrounding this central area of necrosis shows change in the marrow but no evidence of

osteocyte death. There is thickening of the articular cartilage in these cases. Ischaemia of 10 hours was associated with necrosis of the trabeculae in all parts of the epiphysis which were then reabsorbed and replaced by a fibrocartilagenous material. There was considerable deformity of the femoral head. The overlying cartilage is greatly thickened. Similar changes have also been noted by Kemp (1973) and Singleton and Jones (1979).

If the concept of ischaemia of variable duration is accepted as a possible explanation of our histological findings it must be asked how this ischaemia occurs. Is it the result of tamponade due to a small effusion in the presence of active movement (Kemp 1973) or to the leg being held in an extreme position (Henard 1971, Navaro-Quillis and Diaz-Marta 1979). The 'Tamponade theory' will certainly explain the recurrent infarction seen in the Group IV cases, where recurrent episodes of synovitis are commonly seen. However, in Groups II and III cases, where the evidence suggests one episode of ischaemia only with a healing and remodelling process, this theory becomes less attractive. In these cases mechanical deformation of the central necrotic trabeculae could produce repeated infarction by distortion of the vessels within the epiphysis but will not explain the initial episode. Injury to the central branch of the lateral epiphyseal artery (Ferguson 1978), although a possibility, is difficult to explain on a mechanical basis unless there is a localised slip of the growth plate.

Neither the Tamponade nor the positional theories give an explanation for the thickened articular cartilage seen in the uninvolved opposite hip when there is no evidence to suggest ischaemia.

The process of repair

Injury of any type is always followed by a process of repair. In these cases two types of repair are present. In those areas where the trabeculae are necrotic but not crushed the repair process is by creeping substitution (Phemister 1930) in which trabeculae are partially reasorbed after which appositional bone is deposited on the framework of avascular trabeculae. In those areas where the trabeculae are crushed revascularisation of the area is impaired because of recurrent mechanical deformation. The crushed trabecular bone is progressively reabsorbed from its deep surface and replaced by fibrocartilagenous material (Fig. 3.11j). This may be thought of as chondrification of the infarct. Islands of cartilage have been recognised since the reports of Perthes (1913) and Zemansky (1928), but the extent of this tissue in the repair process has not previously been recognised. It is a cellular tissue which is capable of proliferation and is therefore biologically mouldable. Its staining properties are different from the overlying articular cartilage and in this respect, at least, it resembles the matrix in areas of very early cartilage formation in the callus of experimental fractures of the rat metatarsal (Dunham 1978). In fractures this appearance is transient suggesting that in Legg-Calvé-Perthes' disease there may be delay in the maturation of this repair tissue. From research on single and repeated episodes of infarction (Zahir and Freeman 1972, and Sanchis et al 1973), it might be considered that the material might be the consequence of remodelling of the deep part of the thickened articular cartilage. However, this material is only seen in the deep parts of the epiphysis where bone has previously been present. Examination of the serial radiographs suggest it is only in that part of the bony epiphysis which becomes crushed and is reabsorbed that the fibrocartilagenous material is seen.

In the overlying articular cartilage two types of repair process are observed. There is a remodelling process with removal of the articular cartilage from its deep surface and replacement by more cellular fibrocartilage (Fig. 3.11h). This type of repair and remodelling is also seen in the osteoarthritis of adults. In addition, in the thickened articular cartilage endochondral bone formation is observed. This is similar to the changes seen experimentally following infarction of the bony epiphysis (Freeman and England 1969, Kemp 1973). The extent of this change will be proportional to the thickness of the articular cartilage. This is mainly in the anterior and lateral parts of the femoral head with a thin tongue spreading postero-medially.

With regard to treatment the thickened articular cartilage may be considered to be biologically plastic and therefore mouldable during the early phases of the disease. Later the presence of a significant degree of ossification within it will impart rigidity to that part of the femoral head and permit a change of head shape only by subsequent growth and remodelling. This thought may help to explain the different results of containment treatment during the early and late phases of the disease (Lloyd-Roberts et al 1976). In the late phases, where there is established deformity of the femoral head, congruity of the hip joint with the leg in the neutral weight-bearing position will allow better long-term remodelling. Hence containment treatment by varus-rotation osteotomy would be expected to be ineffective as many of the children have an adduction and flexion contracture of the involved hip. In these circumstances re-alignment by an abduction-extension osteotomy would be a more logical procedure to permit long-term remodelling.

REFERENCES

Axhausen G 1923 Der anatomische Krankeitsablauf bei der Koelerschen Krankheit der Metatarsalkopfchen und der Perthesschen Krankheit des Huftkopfes. Archiv für Klinsche Chirurgie 124: 511

Bobechko W, Harris W R 1960 Radiographic density of avascular bone. Journal of Bone and Joint Surgery 42B: 626–632

Burrows H J 1941 Coxa plana with special reference to its pathology and kinship. British Journal of Surgery 29: 23–36

Catterall A 1971 The natural history of Perthes' disease. Journal of Bone and Joint Surgery 53B: 37–53

Catterall A 1981 Legg-Calvé-Perthes' Syndrome. Clinical Orthopaedics and Related Research. 158: 41–52

Catto M 1976 Pathology of aseptic bone necrosis. Aseptic Necrosis of Bone J K Davidson, Exerpta Medica, Amsterdam. p 3–100

Crock H V 1967 The blood supply of the lower limb bones in man. Descriptive and Applied. E & S Livingstone, London.

Dolman C L, Bell H M 1973 The pathology of Legg-Calve-Perthes' disease Journal of Bone and Joint Surgery 55A: 184–188

Dunham J 1978 Cellular biochemistry of undecalcified bone in the response to fracture. Thesis presented for degree of doctor of philosophy in Brunnel University 1978

Edberg E 1918. Studien uber die sogenannten osteochondritis coxae juvenilis Nord. Med. Ark. 51: 63

Ferguson A B 1978 Recent advances in understanding Legg-Perthes' disease Orthopaedic Survey 1: 307–325

Freeman M A R, England J P S 1969 Experimental infarction of the immature canine femoral head. Proceedings of the Royal Society of Medicine 62: 431–433

Gershuni-Gordon D H, Axer A 1974 Synovitis of the hip joint — an experimental model in rabbits. Journal of Bone and Joints Surgery 56B: 69–77

Henard D C 1971 Avascular necrosis of the femoral head in mature and immature dogs. Thesis presented to Committee of Graduate Studies, University of Tenessee, June 1971

Henard D C, Caladruccio R A 1970 Experimental production of roentgenographic and histological changes in the capital femoral epiphysis following abduction extension and internal rotation of the hip. Journal of Bone and Joint Surgery 52A: 600

Inoue A, Ono K 1979 A histological study of idiopathic avascular necrosis of the head of the femur. Journal of Bone and Joint Surgery 61B: 138–143

Jensen O M, Lauritzen J 1976 Legg-Calvé-Perthes' disease — morphological studies in two cases examined at necropsy. Journal of Bone and Joint Surgery 58B: 332–338

Jonaster S 1953. Coxa Plana — a histolo-pathologic and arthrographic study. Acta Orthopaedica Scandinavica Suppl. 12:

Kemp H B S 1973 Perthes' disease: an experimental and clinical study. Annals of Royal College of Surgery of England 52: 18–35

Kemp H B S 1980 Personal communication

Kemp H B S, Boldero J L 1966 Radiological changes in Perthes' disease. British Journal of Radiology 39: 744–760

Lang F J 1932 Osteoarthritis deformans contrasted with osteoarthritis deformans juvenilis. Journal of Bone and Joint Surgery 14: 563–573

Larsen E H, Reiman I 1973 Calvé-Perthes' disease. Acta Orthopaedica Scaninavica 44: 426–438

Lloyd-Roberts G C, Catterall, A, Salamon P B 1976 A controlled study of the indictions and results of femoral osteotomy in Perthes' disease. Journal of Bone and Joint Surgery 58B: 31–36

McKibbin B, Ralis Z 1974 Changes found in a case of Perthes' disease at necropsy. A case report. Journal of Bone and Joint Surgery 56B: 438–447

Mizuno S, Hirayama M, Kotani P T, Simazu A 1966 Pathological histology of the Legg-Calvé-Perthes' disease with a special reference to its experimental production. Medical Journal of Osaka University 17: 177–209

Navaro-Quillis A, Diaz-Marta M A 1979 Study of the blood supply in the ossification of the head of the femur in the rabbit, after postural and pressure change in the joint. Journal of Bone and Joint Surgery 61B: 124

Ogden J A 1974 The changing patterns of proximal femoral vascularity Journal of Bone and Joint Surgery 56A: 941–950

Perthes G C 1913 Osteochondritis deformans juvenilis Archives fur Klinische Chirurgie 101: 779–807

Phemister D B 1921 Operation for epiphysitis of the head of the femur (Perthes' disease) Findings and results. Archives of Surgery 2: 221–230

Phemister D B 1930 Repair of bone in the presence of asceptic necrosis resulting from fractures, transplantations, and vascular obstruction. Journal of Bone and Joint Surgery 12: 769–787

Ponseti I V 1956 Legg-Perthes' disease. Observation on pathological changes in two cases. Journal of Bone and Joint Surgery 38A: 739–750

Reidel G 1922 Beitrag zur pathologischen anatomie de osteochondritis deformans juvenilis Zentralblatt fur Chirurgie 49: 1447–1450

Sanchis M, Zahir A, Freeman M A R 1973 The experimental simulation of Perthes' disease by consecutive interruptions of the blood supply to the capital femoral epiphysis in the puppy. Journal of Bone and Joint Surgery 55A: 335–342

Schwarz E 1914 quoted by Edgren W. Acta Orthopaedica Scandinavica Supp. 84: 25

Singleton W B, Jones E L 1979 The experimental induction of subclinical Perthes' disease in the puppy following arthrotomy and intracapsular tamponade. Journal of Comparative Pathology and Therapeutics 89: 57–71

Trueta J 1957 The normal vascular anatomy of the femoral head during growth Journal of Bone and Joint Surgery 39B: 358–394

Zahir A, Freeman M A R 1972 Cartilage changes following a single episode of infarction of the capital femoral epiphysis in the dog. Journal of Bone and Joint Surgery 54A: 215–136

Zemansky A P 1928 The pathology and pathogenesis of Legg-Calve-Perthes' disease (Osteochondritis juvenilis deformans coxae) American Journal of Surgery 4: 169–184

4

Clinical features

Although ultimately Legg-Calvé-Perthes' disease will be diagnosed as the result of radiographs taken of a child presenting with hip symptoms, there are a number of important clinical features of this condition which will be helpful not only in diagnosis but also in management.

Age and sex

It is generally accepted that this condition is more common in boys who also have a better long term prognosis than girls. In the 1970 survey of 388 cases collected from many centres in the British Isles I found the average age of onset was approximately six years with a span of 22 months to 13 years (Fig. 4.1); 305 of these cases (82 per cent)

had an age of onset between the age of four and nine years at the time of presentation. In contrast to a number of previous reports, in this series the average age of onset for girls was younger than that for boys (Table 4.1), the sex ratio was 3.67:1 which corresponds to previous series.

Bilateral cases

These cases differ from the rest of the survey, having a younger age of onset and a much greater preponderence of boys with a ratio of 7:1. Girls again showed a younger age of onset (Tables 4.1 and 4.2). This confirms the thoughts already discussed in the chapter on aetiology, that in bilateral disease the underlying abnormality becomes more

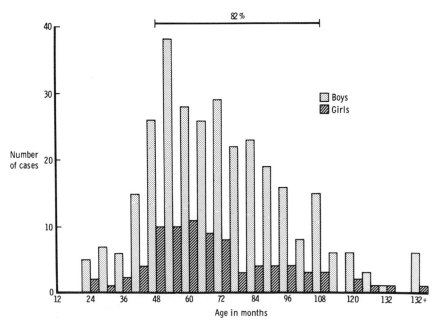

Fig. 4.1 Histogram of age at preservation

Table 4.1 Sex ratio (1970 survey)

	Number	Ratio
All cases	388	3.67:1
Unilateral cases	248	3.30:1
Bilateral cases	65	7.1 :1
Group I	30	14 :1
Group II	143	3.7 :1
Group III	108	2.3 :1
Group IV	43	2.9 :1

Table 4.2 Age at presentation (1970 survey)

	Number	Age Average in months
All cases	388	71.75 ± 24.9
Boys	305	72.7 ± 25.1
Girls	83	70.34 ± 25.4
Bilateral cases	65	68.7 ± 24.5
Boys	57	69.0 ± 24.7
Girls	8	65.0 ± 24.4

apparent with the younger age of onset and increased incidence of associated anomalies. Girls have a lower frequency of disease but a younger age of onset with a more serious outlook in the long term.

Presentation

This condition may be diagnosed as a result of acute or chronic symptoms. The acute symptoms are part of the irritable hip syndrome. In the chronic presentation, aching commonly felt in the hip, thigh or knee and associated with stiffness and limp may be the presenting features.

Acute presentation

The irritable hip syndrome

This syndrome sometimes referred to as 'transient synovitis' was first noted by Lovett and Morse (1892) and subsequently considered in detail by Todd (1925) and Fairbank (1926). It is more common in the Spring and Summer months and affects boys more commonly than girls. The onset of pain felt in the groin or knee is usually sudden and frequently at night. Commonly, therefore, these children are unable to get out of bed and take weight on the leg in the morning.

Clinical examination reveals no wasting but a

few degrees of fixed flexion in the hip and limitation of abduction of the flexed hip. There is loss of internal rotation, particularly with the hip in flexion.

The radiographic appearances, which will be considered in detail in Chapter 5, are essentially normal although in 50 per cent there is an increase in the infero-medial joint space (Anderson and Stewart 1970). Approximately half the children have a mild pyrexia and 20 per cent have a raised E.S.R.

Clinical course

In the great majority of cases these symptoms settle within a few days with simple rest in bed. In a small percentage of cases symptoms may persist for up to two weeks. Should irritability persist longer than approximately ten days the child may require admission to hospital for assessment and traction. On this regime persistent symptoms which do not resolve with a short period of traction should be regarded as an indiction for aspiration of the hip.

Various reports, Spock (1959), Jacobs (1960), Adams (1963) and Valderrama (1963), state that between 1 and 7 per cent of children with an irritable hip syndrome subsequently develop Perthes' disease. However, in some cases established changes of the condition are seen radiologically on the initial radiographs taken at the time of hip irritability.

In the long term follow-up of the irritable hip syndrome Valderrama (1963) has reported a high incidence of coxa magna with or without changes of osteoarthritis. This abnormality appeared to be confined to children with symptoms starting over the age of eight years. Minor degrees of coxa magna and broadening of the femoral head were seen in adults who had had an irritable hip under this age.

Differential diagnosis

Acute and chronic infection may present with an identical clinical syndrome as may rheumatic fever. In this latter condition, however, the arthritis is usually passing from one joint to another in the course of several days. In addition, a precordial murmur may be heard in many cases; the E.S.R. is raised above 20 mm in the first hour and the anti-streptolycin titre levels are also elevated.

Delayed or chronic presentation

In the British Isles this is the commonest presentation with pain, stiffness and a limp.

a. Pain

This is commonly mild and described as an ache in the groin and anterior thigh but may only be felt in the knee. It is usually worse after rest and on getting out of bed in the morning. It is troublesome in the evening after exercise. It seldom disturbs sleep.

b. Stiffness

This is usually most marked in the morning, after rest and in the evening.

c. Limp

This is nearly always noticed as an early symptom and is most marked in the morning and following games. The families usually state that the child, who has normally been an extremely active person, starts to tire more easily and, particularly, refuses to walk long distances.

General health

All these children are usually in good general health but it is not uncommon for the symptoms already discussed and described to become more apparent first after either a mild upper respiratory tract infection or one of the childhood illnesses such as measles.

Past history and family history

Details of previous illnesses and operations should be carefully enquired into, particularly for the repair of an inguinal hernia or any history suggestive of genito-urinary abnormality (Catterall et al 1971). A similar history should also be sought in the parents and first degree relatives.

Clinical examination

A thorough clinical examination should be made of all these children and their height and weight noted. In particular signs in other joints to suggest a multiple epiphyseal dypslasia should be looked for and noted. Any abnormalities of the hands, particularly short phalanges, should raise the question of a Perthes-like change. During examination the changes of juvenile myxoedema should be looked for. These are a dry skin, obesity, constipation and delayed reflexes. The presence or absence of inguinal herniae and undescended testicle or hypospadias should also be noted.

Gait

An abnormality of gait is present in almost all these children. The limp in the early stages is of the antalgic type in which the child walks with a stiff hip favouring the involved leg. As the disease progresses there is often the development of fixed deformity of both adduction and flexion. This produces a characteristic gait of the dipping short leg type and a short stride on the involved side.

With the child lying at rest on the couch apparent shortening of the involved leg will be noted together with wasting which is mainly above the knee and of the buttock, but may occasionally involve the calf as well. The presence of apparent shortening is due to a combination of fixed adduction and flexion. These signs should be carefully looked for and noted using the Thomas' test. From the position of fixed deformity the hip usually flexes to approximately a right angle but it is noted that the leg is usually in external rotation. With the leg in extension the range of abduction, adduction, and internal rotation are reduced compared with the opposite side.

The feet and subtaloid joints should be examined. Stiffness in the subtaloid joint is noted in approximately 20 per cent of cases with Legg-Calvé-Perthes' disease and radiographs may reveal the changes of Köhler's disease. In the absence of radiographic evidence of Köhler's disease stiffness of the subtaloid joint may be an early sign of Still's disease or juvenile rheumatoid arthritis.

Follow-up examinations

At the time of each follow-up examination the patient's height and weight should be noted. It is not unusual for these children to grow very little during the active phase of the disease. The subsequent growth spurt will restore this deficit in the younger child but not always in the older age groups.

Either following femoral osteotomy or in the follow-up of cases in which no specific treatment is advised clinical examination is important. The earliest clinical sign of healing is an increase in the range of movement of the hip first seen in the range of abduction and subsequently in the range of internal rotation. During the active phase of the disease progressive stiffness of the hip joint or loss of abduction and internal rotation leading to adduction contracture should be viewed with apprehension as progressive deformity of the femoral head is commonly seen in those cases in which fixed deformity is present. The presence of these clinical signs suggest that the hip is 'at risk' (Ch. 7).

Investigation

All children presenting with the acute or chronic syndromes described above require investigations to exclude: acute or chronic infection, acetabular dysplasia, minor degrees of slipped epiphysis. Gauchers' disease, eosinophylic granuloma, multiple epiphyseal dysplasia, cretinism, and lymphomas.

The major investigation will obviously be radiographic and the changes observed will be considered in detail in Chapter 5. All cases, however, should have a full blood count including white cell differential and E.S.R. together with routine testing of the urine. An I.V.P. is indicated in those cases in which there is any suggestion of a renal anomaly, the presence of a urinary infection, particularly in boys, and changes suggestive of posterior Group I Perthes' disease (Ch. 5).

Bone scan

In recent years a number of investigators (Ash et al 1976, Dahigelis 1975, Fisher et al 1980, Sutherland et al 1980) have used isotope imaging of the hip joints in the diagnosis and assessment of Legg-Calvé-Perthes' disease. Although some rather extravagant claims are made for this investigation it would seem to be of value in two instances. Firstly, in those cases of the acute irritable hip syndrome in which symptoms fail to settle in two or three weeks. Sutherland et al (1980) has reported that while the majority of children in these circumstances have a normal bone scan, in those cases destined to develop Legg-Calvé-Perthes' disease a lytic triangle or cold spot is seen as a wedge in the lateral aspect of the hip joint. This change preceded those seen radiologically by several weeks. Secondly, Danigelis et al (1975) have used imaging during the established phase of the disease to demonstrate the degree of involvement of the epiphysis and onset of the healing and revascularisation stage. These findings have also been confirmed by Tachdjian (1980). It is, however, the author's experience that, in the established disease, unless very good quality pictures can be obtained the results tend to be rather inconclusive. The great place of radio-imaging would seem to be in the differential diagnosis of those cases of the irritable hip syndrome in which symptoms persist and the question of early Legg-Calvé-Perthes' disease has to be excluded. It may also prove to be of value in establishing when the healing phase of the disease is occurring.

REFERENCES

Adams J A 1963 Transient synovitis of the hip found in children. Journal of Bone and Joint Surgery 45B: 471–476
Anderson J, Stewart A M, 1970 The significance of the magnitude of the medial hip space. British Journal of Radiology 43: 238–239
Ash J M, Gilday D L, Reilly B J, 1975 Pinhole imaging of hip disorders in children. Journal of Nuclear Medicine 16: 512–513

Catterall A, Lloyd-Roberts G C, Wynne-Davies R 1971
  Association of Perthes' disease with congenital anomalies of
  genito-urinary tract and inguinal region. Lancet i: 996–997
Danigelis J A, Fisher R L, Ozonoff M B, Sziklas J J 1975
  99mTC-Polyphosphate bone imaging in Legg-Perthes' disease.
  Radiology Vol: 115 2: 407–413
Fairbank H A T 1926 Discussion of non-tuberculous coxitis in
  the young. British Medical Journal ii: 828
Fisher R L, Roderique J Q, Brown D C, Danigelis J A,
  Ozonff M B, Sziklas J J 1980 The relationship of osotopic
  bone imaging findings to prognosis in Legg-Perthes' disease.
  Clinical Orthopaedics and Related Research 150: 23–29
Jacob B W, 1960 Early recognition of osteochondrosis of the
  capital epiphysis of the femur. Journal of the American
  Medical Association 172: 527

Lovett R W, Morse J L 1892 A transient or ephemeral form of
  hip disease, with a report of cases. Boston Medical and
  Surgical Journal 127: 161
Spock A 1959 Transient synovitis of the hip found in children.
  Pediatrics 24: 1042
Sutherland A D, Savage J P, Paterson D C, Foster B K 1980
  The nuclide bone scan in the diagnosis and management of
  Perthes' disease. Journal of Bone and Joint Surgery
  62B: 300–306
Tachdjian M O 1980 Personal communication
Todd A H 1925 Discussion on the differential diagnosis of
  non-tuberculous coxitis in children and adolescence.
  Proceedings of the Royal Society of Medicine18: 31
Valderrama J A F de 1963 The observation hip syndrome and
  its sequelae Journal of Bone and Joint Surgery 45B: 462–470

5

Radiological features

INTRODUCTION

From a clinical point of view it is difficult to separate true Legg-Calvé-Perthes' disease from those conditions producing a Perthes-like change. However, careful examination of the radiographs will usually allow a positive diagnosis of this condition and also separate it from those conditions which will produce a Perthes-like change. The importance of good quality radiographs cannot be overestimated. In order that these may be obtained the hip should be as mobile as possible, and this may only be achieved in some cases after a short spell of traction. The views required are antero-posterior radiographs of the hips with the hip in the neutral position together with Lauenstein lateral views (Fig. 5.1a, b). Views of the hands, wrists and feet will establish bone age and the co-existence of Köhler's disease. The 'frog' lateral views taken when there is still marked restriction of abduction and flexion produce an appearance which is often difficult to interpret. In addition to these radiographs, views of the knees, spine and skull may be required to exclude the other causes of a Perthes-like change.

The differential diagnosis of Perthes-like change

There are a number of conditions which may be confused radiologically with Legg-Calvé-Perthes' disease. Clinically many of these are indistinguishable and are only separated on their radiological appearances. It is useful to consider this differential diagnosis in those conditions which are associated with unilateral and bilateral changes (Table 5.1).

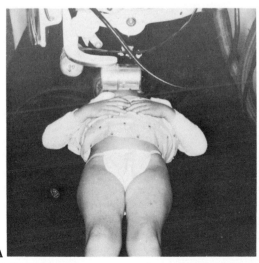
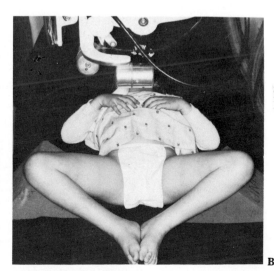

A   **B**

Fig. 5.1 Positions for (a) antero-posterior and (b) Lauenstein lateral radiographs of the hip joint.

Table 5.1 Differential diagnosis of a Perthes-like change

Bilateral changes	Unilateral changes
Hypothyroidism	Infection Gauchers disease
Spondylo-epiphyseal dysplasia	Eosinophilic granuloma Lymphoma
Multiple epiphyseal dysplasia	Sickle cell disease Haemophilia

Table 5.2 (After Crossan 1980)

		Bilateral Legg-Calve-Perthes' disease	Hypothyroidism	Spondylo-epiphyseal dysplasia	Multiple epiphyseal dysplasia
Femoral capital epiphysis	Development	Not delayed	Delayed	Delayed	Delayed
	Changes	Asymmetrical	Symmetrical	Symmetrical	Symmetrical
	Appearance	Irregular areas of increased density and re-absorption	Small irregular density	Low cresentic	Multiple ossification centres
Metaphysis		Involved	Wide	Uninvolved but cup-shaped	Uninvolved but cup-shaped
Acetabulum		Adaptive changes particularly under age of 6 years	Normal	Fluffy outline to roof	Fluffy outline to roof
Spine		Normal	Normal	Platyspondyly	Normal
Body proportions		Normal	Normal	Short trunk	Normal/short limbs

Bilateral changes

Crossan (1980) has recently studied the conditions associated with failure of normal development of the upper femoral epiphysis and has discussed their differential diagnosis (Table 5.2). The main difficulty is to separate the changes associated with bilateral Legg-Calvé-Perthes' disease, hypothyroidism, multiple epiphyseal dysplasia (Fig. 5.2) and spondylo-epiphyseal dysplasia tarda. The importance of separating these conditions from true Legg-Calvé-Perthes' disease cannot be over-emphasised. This is because they do not follow the same natural history and particularly do not respond to treatment in the same way.

Unilateral changes

There are a number of conditions which may simulate unilateral Perthes' disease. These include infection, Gaucher's disease, eosinophilic granuloma, lymphoma, sickle-cell disease, and haemophilia.

1. Infection. A Perthes-like change may be seen following either acute or chronic infection of the hip joint (Figs. 5.3, 5.4). The infection may occur either following an acute septic arthritis or as a consequence of osteomyelitis in the femoral neck. It is presumed that the infection produces pressure or even thrombosis in the vessels supplying the epiphysis and infarction of bone occurs following this. Tuberculosis may present with a localised osteolytic area in the femoral neck leading to a premature growth arrest with subsequent femoral head deformity.

2. Gaucher's disease. Deposits of Gaucher's material are classically seen in the femoral neck in

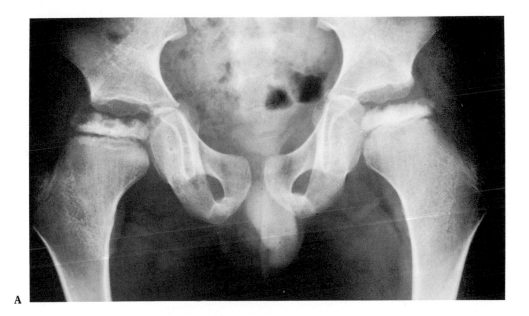

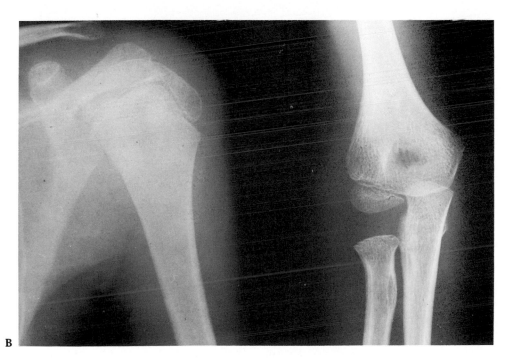

Fig. 5.2 Multiple epiphyseal dysplasia. (a) Child aged 6 years presenting with a Perthes-like change. Note the symmetrical bilateral changes with a long femoral neck. (b) The shoulders and elbows from this case.

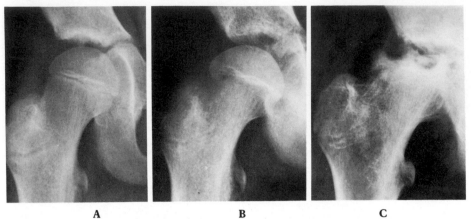

A	**B**	**C**

Fig. 5.3 Infection producing a Perthes-like change. (a) July 1978. Child aged 10 years with symptoms of acute suprative arthritis of the left hip joint. The hip was decompressed by open operation. (b) August 1978. Reabsorption of the lateral aspect of the femoral neck and increased density of the epiphysis with widening of the inferomedial joint space. (c) November 1979. Established Perthes-like changes.

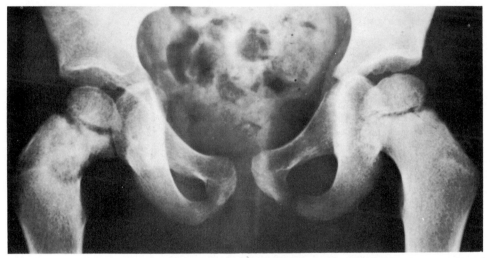

Fig. 5.4 Radiograph of a child presenting with a tuberculous lesion in the femoral neck and a Perthes-like change (Dr Murray's case).

this condition. This may lead to either a pathological fracture of the neck producing an appearance suggestive of coxa vara or to a Perthes-like change in the upper femoral epiphysis (Fig. 5.5). Radiologically, in addition to the abnormality in the femoral neck there is a failure of remodelling, particularly of the supracondylar region of the lower femur. Clinically these children present with anaemia, thrombocytopaenia, and have enlargement of both liver and spleen.

3. Eosinophilic granuloma. This condition may present with a painful hip, and radiological deposits in the femoral neck. A Perthes-like change may subsequently develop. Other lesions may be apparent on the hip radiographs in the pelvis or on a skeletal survey. A blood count may or may not reveal an eosinophilia. The E.S.R. is usually raised.

4. Lymphoma. Deposits of lymphomatous and other material (Fig. 5.4) can occur not only in the femoral neck but also in the subtrochanteric regions of the femur. Those situated in the femoral neck may or may not be associated with changes reminiscent of Legg-Calvé-Perthes' disease, the infarction is usually complete, and the changes progressive.

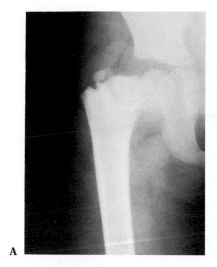
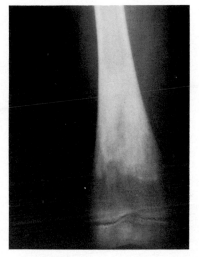

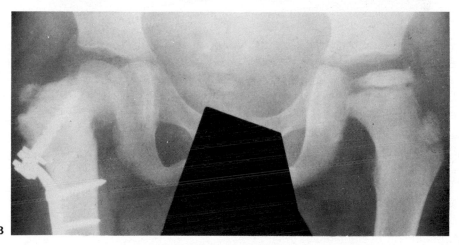

Fig. 5.5 Gaucher's disease. (a) February 1979. Child aged 3 years 6 months with known Gaucher's disease who presented with a pathological fracture of the right femoral neck. The increased density and absence of remodelling in the lower femur may be noted. (b) June 1979. Following internal fixation of the fracture of the femoral neck a Perthes-like change is observed in the left hip.

Radiological features of the irritable hip syndrome

Although in the majority of cases radiographs taken during the acute stage of this syndrome are normal, two radiological signs were found to be of value. These are an increase in the inferomedial joint space and an alteration in the capsular shadow on the lateral aspect of the hip joint. These factors have both been discussed in detail by Jansen (1923) and Ferguson (1954). Anderson and Stewart (1970) states that more than half the children with an irritable hip have an increase in the inferomedial joint space and that these children do not subsequently develop progressive changes.

LEGG-CALVÉ-PERTHES' DISEASE

Although Legg (1910), Calvé (1910), Perthes (1910) and Waldenström (1909), each individually described the radiological features of this condition it is due to the extensive writings of Waldenström, 1920, 1934, 1938, that credit should be given for a detailed discussion of the early diagnostic signs and particularly the staging of the disease in its natural history. In practice the radiological problems are firstly to establish the diagnosis in the early phase, secondly the extent of epiphyseal involvement and thirdly the staging of the disease. These factors will be considered separately.

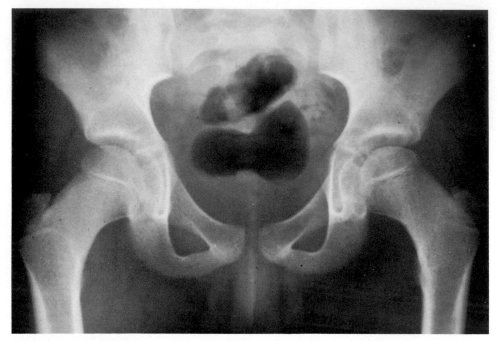

Fig. 5.6 Child aged 7 years presenting with the signs of the Irritable Hip Syndrome of the left hip. The antero-posterior radiographs show a wide inferomedial joint space and a small epiphysis. He subsequently developed Legg-Calvé-Perthes' disease.

Early diagnosis

Although many signs have been described four signs are of value.

1. Lateral displacement of the femoral head.
2. A subchondral fracture line.
3. Increased epiphyseal density.
4. The size of the epiphyseal nucleus.

1. Lateral displacement of the femoral head

This sign, initially described by Waldenström (1920), is an increase in the distance between the medial margin of the metaphysis and the tear drop of the acetabulum, and is present in many cases at an early stage (Fig. 5.6). Caffey (1968) found it in 26 of 30 cases, while Kemp and Boldero (1966) noted it as an early sign in 80 per cent. Anderson and Stewart (1970) noted its presence in 75 per cent of their patients but added that it was also noted in 50 per cent of children with an irritable hip, the appearances subsequently returning to normal.

2. A subchondral fracture line

It is difficult to be certain who first described this sign. Waldenström (1938) comments on an osteoporotic area in the subchondral zone of the epiphysis. Burrows (1941, 1954) noted subchondral fissures while Caffey (1968) discussed the sign in detail noting the appearances of intra-epiphyseal gas in association with these fractures. More recently Salter and Thompson (1980) have related the prognosis in the long term to the extent of the fracture line, a fact also noted by Catterall in his discussion of the Groups (1971, 1981).

The subchondral fracture line is an early sign in this disease. It is best observed on the Lauenstein lateral view (Fig. 5.7). It starts at the anterior margin of the epiphysis passing posteriorly in the subchondral zone. It is unfortunate, however, that it is present only transiently in the early phases of the disease and is only therefore of value in management in 25 per cent of cases.

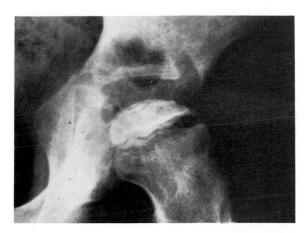

Fig. 5.7 The subchondral fracture line. Lateral radiograph of a child with Group III Legg-Calvé-Perthes' disease showing the subchondral fracture line reaching into the posterior third of the epiphysis.

3. Increased epiphyseal density

This is a variable sign (Fig. 5.8a, see p. 46) For the most part it is the radiological manifestation of apositional new bone formation being laid on the framework of avascular trabeculae (Bobechko and Harris 1960). Dolman and Bell (1973) comment that the necrotic marrow becomes calcified increasing the sclerosis in the central part of the epiphysis. Localised sclerosis in the dome of the epiphysis is seen in association with crushing of the trabeculae and is again a feature of the early phases. Waldenström (1934) noted that in some cases the sclerosis affects the anterior part of the epiphysis.

4. The size of the epiphyseal nucleus

Both Caffey (1968) and Jacobs (1976) note that a small epiphyseal nucleus is seen in approximately 50 per cent of cases. This in part accounts for the increase in the inferomedial joint space (Fig. 5.6).

The stages of the disease and its natural history

Many authors have discussed the radiological course of this disease, Waldenström (1923) describes four phases (Fig. 5.8). There is an Initial phase which is subdivided into the phases of Onset and Fragmentation in which the femoral head is liable to become deformed. This is followed by a phase of Healing, the duration of which can extend to up to two years. During this time ossification of the biologically deformed femoral head occurs. The third phase, the Growing period, is a major remodelling process which ultimately leads to the Definitive period which may or may not be complicated by a degenerative arthritis. A number of other workers confirm these findings and produced minor modifications in the radiological course (Jonaster 1953).

Somerville (1971) regarded the initial phase as ischaemic and associated it with sclerosis. This was followed by a phase of fragmentation which he felt was better considered as a phase of reabsorption of the involved epiphysis. The third period was followed by a phase of healing during which reossification of the epiphysis occurred. The final phase of remodelling continued until the end of growth.

The extent of epiphyseal involvement

It has been an assumption of the majority of previous reports that the ischaemic process involved the whole epiphysis. This suggests that the prognosis is therefore influenced by such factors as the age and sex of the patient, the stage of the disease at diagnosis and the nature of treatment but not by the extent of the initial ischaemia. O'Garra (1959) was the first to report half head Perthes' disease in which only the anterior part of the epiphysis was involved although Waldenström (1934) had noted that the sclerosis might only be confined to the anterior part of the epiphysis. Ralston (1961) also related the degree of radiological involvement to the final outcome. Catterall (1970, 1971, 1981) pursued the concept of half head Perthes' disease, subdividing the process into four separate groups dependant on the degree of radiological involvement. He showed that the prognosis was proportional to the degree of radiological involvement of the epiphysis. These Groups can be recognised in the early stages and do not change during the course of the disease.

The Groups

Before considering the Groups in detail it is important to realise that the clinician is trying to make an assessment of the degree of radiological

Fig. 5.8 The stages of Legg-Calvé-Perthes' disease. This child was aged 7 years 8 months at the time of the diagnosis. Treatment — a weight-relieving caliper.

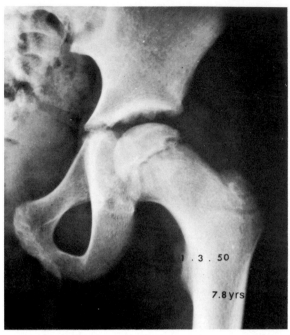

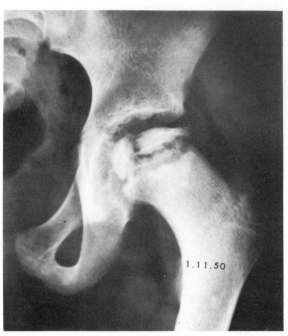

Fig. 5.8(a) March 1950. The phase of onset. Antero-posterior radiographs showing the increased epiphyseal density and widening of the inferomedial joint space.

Fig. 5.8(b) November 1950. The phase of fragmentation. The lateral two-thirds of the epiphysis is collapsed and is being reabsorbed with an intact medial fragment (Group III). There is lateral uncovering of the femoral head.

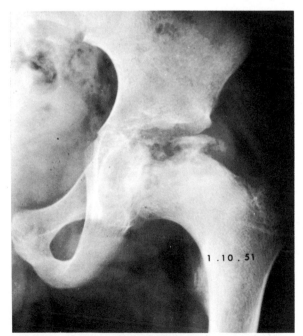

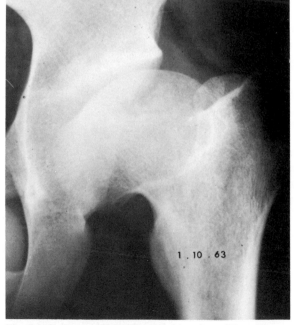

Fig. 5.8(c) October 1951. The phase of healing. Healing is established with considerable deformity of the femoral head. There is an increase in size of the medial segment and in the size and quality of the bone forming laterally.

Fig. 5.8(d) October 1963. The definitive phase. There is a coxa magna with deformity of the femoral head. Poor result. The femoral neck is short and the greater trochanter relatively high.

involvement of the epiphysis by the use of good quality radiographs taken in the antero-posterior and Lauenstein lateral positions (Fig. 5.1). This assessment is made by reference to the presence or absence of a number of radiological signs, some of which have already been considered (Table 5.3 and 5.4). A number of the signs are present early in the disease while others are only present in the established stage. In particular the subchondral fracture line is an excellent sign in the early stages but is unfortunately in only approximately 25 per cent of cases.

Group I

Figure 5.9a (see over) is a drawing of the radiological features of this Group in which only the anterior part of the epiphysis is involved. It differs from the other groups to be discussed in that no collapse occurs and no sequestrum is seen. On the antero-posterior radiograph (Fig. 5.10 see over) the epiphysis has a somewhat sclerotic appearance but its height is maintained. A lytic area or defect may be observed either centrally or superiorly in the dome of the epiphysis. The lateral radiograph shows that the defect seen on the antero-posterior view is in the subchondral zone usually centrally but it may be anterior or posterior. In every case, however, there is a tongue of normal epiphysis reaching the anterior margin of the growth plate (Fig. 5.10b). As the course of the disease is followed radiologically it is observed that the defect tends to deepen for a number of months as the surrounding epiphysis continues to grow and then slowly fills in by ossification occurring from the periphery of the defect. Herring et al (1980) has commented in detail on the site of this defect, considering it to be due to an abnormality of blood supply. Catterall (1970) has observed the presence of posterior involvement and has found a strong correlation with this site and the presence of genito-urinary disease; a Group I case with defects situated posteriorly, therefore, would be regarded as indication for an intravenous pylogram. The benign course of this disease has been emphasised by Blakemore and Harrison (1979).

Table 5.3 Epiphyseal signs

| | Group | | | |
	I	II	III	IV
Sequestrum	No	Yes	Yes	Yes
Sub-chondral Fracture line	No	Anterior half	Posterior half	Posterior margin
Junction involved/uninvolved segments	Clear	Clear 'V' or vertical	Sclerotic in posterior third	Nil
Viable epiphysis on growth plate	Anterior margin	Anterior half	Posterior half	Nil
Triangular appearance to medial/lateral sides of epiphysis	No	No	Occasional	In early stages

Table 5.4 Metaphyseal signs

| | Group | | | |
	I	II	III	IV
Metaphyseal Reaction	No	Localised antero-lateral	Diffuse or anterior	Diffuse or central
Posterior Remodelling	No	No	No	Yes

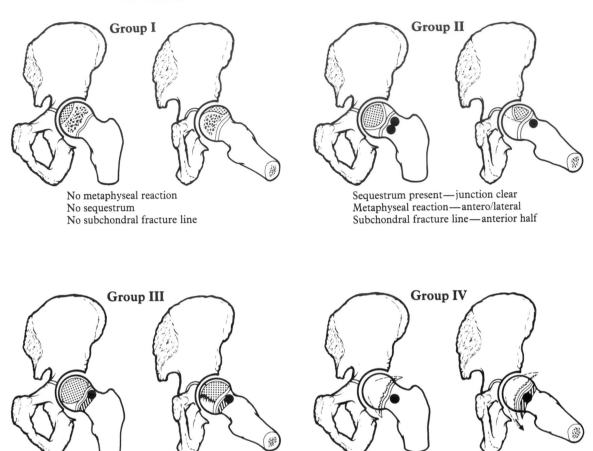

Group I

No metaphyseal reaction
No sequestrum
No subchondral fracture line

Group II

Sequestrum present—junction clear
Metaphyseal reaction—antero/lateral
Subchondral fracture line—anterior half

Group III

Sequestrum — large — junction sclerotic
Metaphyseal reaction — diffuse antero/lateral area
Subchondral fracture line — posterior half

Group IV

Whole head involvement
Metaphyseal reaction — central or diffuse
Posterior remodelling

Fig. 5.9 Drawings of Groups I to IV

Group II

In this variety rather more of the anterior part of
the epiphysis is involved (Fig. 5.9b). Radiologically the main difference in the course of the disease
is that the involved segment, after a phase of reabsorption, undergoes collapse with the formation of
a dense collapsed segment or sequestrum. In the
early phases (Figs. 5.11, 5.12) the area of reabsorption is seen in the anterior part of the epiphysis and continues right up to its anterior margin.
There may be a subchondral fracture line but this
only involves the anterior half of the epiphysis. In
the established case on the antero-posterior radiograph the sequestrum appears as a dense overall
mass with viable fragments on the medial and

lateral side (Figs. 5.11, 5.12 see page 49 and 50).
When collapse of the epiphysis occurs, the variable fragment will maintain its height. On the
lateral radiograph the sequestrum is separated
posteriorly from the viable fragments by a 'V'
which when present is characteristic of this Group
(Fig. 5.12a, b). On occasions, however, the junction is less well defined, being either vertical or
sloping posteriorly (Fig. 5.11a). In either case,
however, a tongue of viable epiphysis is always
seen reaching well forward along the anterior half
of the growth plate. If there is a metaphyseal lesion this is usually a well defined cyst situated in
the central or lateral part of the metaphysis on the
antero-posterior radiograph. It is always anterior

Fig. 5.10 Group I. Child aged 4 years 7 months at the time of diagnosis. No treatment.

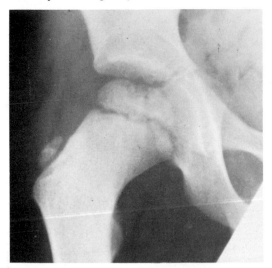 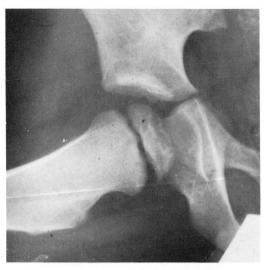

Fig. 5.10(a) March 1964. Antero-posterior radiographs showing a defect in the superior part of the epiphysis. The lateral radiograph confirms the Group I appearance with the defect situated centrally. Normal textured epiphysis reaches the anterior margin of the growth plate.

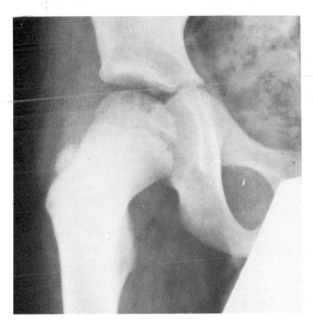 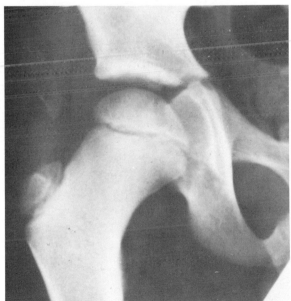

Fig. 5.10(b) August 1964. Healing is well established.

(c) June 1966. Healed. Good result.

in the lateral view. It is transitory and disappears with healing.

The course of the disease is that the involved collapsed segment is progressively removed producing the appearance of fragmentation, following which, regeneration by ossification of the involved area occurs from the periphery of the subsequent defect (Fig. 5.12c, d).

Group III

In this variety only a small portion of the epiphysis remains uninvolved (Fig. 5.9c). On the antero-posterior radiograph during the early phases of the disease a subchondral fracture line is observed situated in the dome of the epiphysis, producing the appearance of a 'head within a head'. On the

Fig. 5.11 Group II. Child aged 4 years 10 months at diagnosis. No treatment.

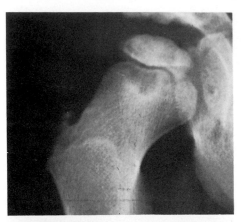

Fig. 5.11(a) August 1957. Antero-posterior radiograph. There is a central area of reabsorption with good medial and lateral segments. There is a central metaphyseal lesion. Lateral radiograph: the changes are confined to the anterior part of the epiphysis only. The metaphyseal lesion is anterior under the involved segment.

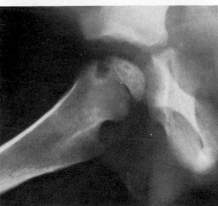

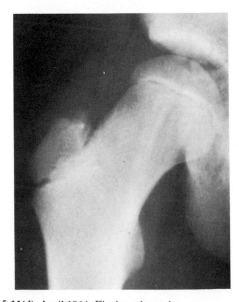

Fig. 5.11(b) March 1958. There is now a central sequestrum with good medial and lateral segments.

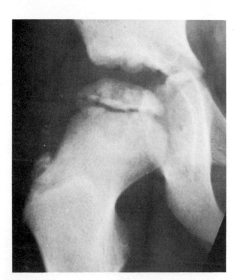

Fig. 5.11(c) June 1968. Healing is well established with reabsorption of the dense central segment.

Fig. 5.11(d) April 1964. Final result good.

Fig. 5.12 Group II. Child aged 4 years at the time of diagnosis. No treatment.

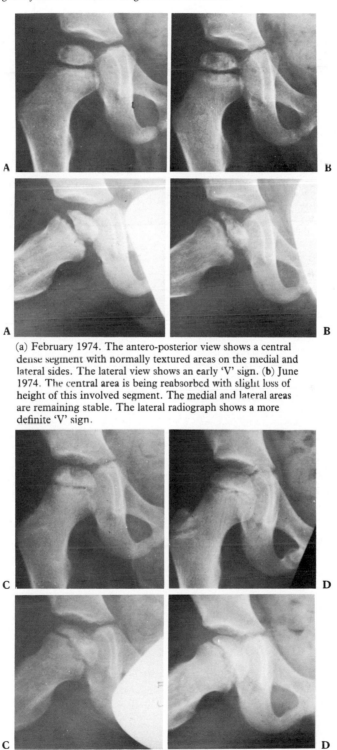

(a) February 1974. The antero-posterior view shows a central dense segment with normally textured areas on the medial and lateral sides. The lateral view shows an early 'V' sign. (b) June 1974. The central area is being reabsorbed with slight loss of height of this involved segment. The medial and lateral areas are remaining stable. The lateral radiograph shows a more definite 'V' sign.

(c) Healing is well established.   (d) Healed with good final result.

Fig. 5.13 Group III. Child aged 7 years at diagnosis. Treatment — prolonged bed rest.

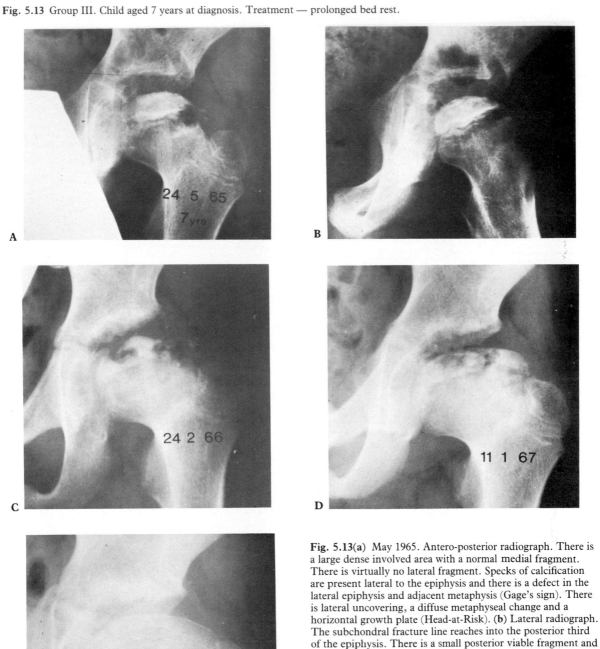

Fig. 5.13(a) May 1965. Antero-posterior radiograph. There is a large dense involved area with a normal medial fragment. There is virtually no lateral fragment. Specks of calcification are present lateral to the epiphysis and there is a defect in the lateral epiphysis and adjacent metaphysis (Gage's sign). There is lateral uncovering, a diffuse metaphyseal change and a horizontal growth plate (Head-at-Risk). **(b)** Lateral radiograph. The subchondral fracture line reaches into the posterior third of the epiphysis. There is a small posterior viable fragment and a sclerotic junction between the involved and uninvolved areas. There is a diffuse metaphyseal lesion with an anterior defect.

Fig. 5.13(c) February 1966. Involved area is becoming reabsorbed and there is further loss of height of the epiphysis. The medial fragment remains viable and is beginning to increase in size. **(d)** January 1967. Healing is now established, a mass of new bone is beginning to form laterally in the area of the previous specks of calcification.

Fig. 5.13(e) October 1969. Healed. Result poor.

lateral radiograph the subchondral fracture line is seen preceding from the anterior margin of the epiphysis into its posterior part and may be used to delineate the junction between the involved and uninvolved segments (Fig. 5.13b). This view will also show that only a small portion of the posterior part of the head is uninvolved. In contrast to Group II the junction of the sequestrum with the viable segments is often not clearly definable, the two blending in an area of sclerosis. In subsequent radiographs there is a large collapsed sequestrum centrally placed with normally textured segments on the medial and lateral side. The segment on the medial side is often of reasonable size but on the lateral side it is often so small and osteoporitic that it is difficult to recognise. Just lateral to the epiphysis in many cases are specks of calcification. These have been shown in the Chapter on the Morbid Anatomy to be ossification occurring in the enlarged cartilagenous part of the femoral head.

Metaphyscal changes are usually generalised in this Group. They take two forms, firstly a generalised reaction situated through the metaphyseal region producing a widening of the growth plate. Secondly, there may or may not be an associated anterior lesion similar to that seen in Group II. It is generally accepted that an extensive metaphyseal lesion is commonly associated with a poor result.

The course of the disease is essentially similar to that in Group II (Figs. 5.13, 5.14). When collapse of the epiphysis occurs it is onto the height of the posterior and medial fragment (Fig. 5.14). Because of the difference in the height of the posterior viable fragments in Groups II and III collapse will be more marked in the Group III cases producing a greater degree of femoral head deformity. The sequestrum so formed is gradually reabsorbed after which regeneration by re-ossification begins from the periphery of the defect. At this stage the calcification, noticed initially lateral to the epiphysis in the early stages, starts to enlarge forming a well-defined mass of ossification which may spread as a surrounding shell on the posterior and medial sides of the epiphysis (Fig. 5.14c).

Many people have difficulty in separating Group II from Group III disease. This is because they represent a common morphological process. De-spite this, however, it is important to try and separate the two as in the long term they carry a very different form of prognosis and the clear cut examples of each may bias the clinician for or against the definitive forms of treatment which he may be considering.

Group IV

In this variety, a drawing of which is seen in Fig. 5.9d, the whole epiphysis is involved. On the antero-posterior radiograph total collapse of the epiphysis produces a dense line and there is an early loss of height between the growth plate and the roof of the acetabulum indicating flattening of the femoral head. By contrast with the previous Groups the deformation of the femoral head is not only anterior and lateral but also posterior and medial producing a 'mushroom' type of appearance. Posteriorly this may be seen as remodelling of the posterior metaphysis, usually straight. This 'beaking' is similar to that seen in the remodelling phase of a slipped epiphysis (Fig. 5.15a, b).

In the early phases of this Group there are some incidences in which the radiological appearances are difficult to interpret and separate from those seen in Group I. The characteristic radiological sign in these circumstances is a triangular shape to both the medial and lateral aspects of the epiphysis seen on the antero-posterior radiograph (Fig. 5.15a). Also, examination of the lateral radiograph will show that the changes involve the whole of the epiphysis and not just the anterior part as seen in Group I. In the younger age group a globular epiphysis is often seen which then fails to enlarge. Subsequently ossification is observed as a linear line along the growth plate (Fig. 5.15a). With time the original epiphysis may or may not collapse but then is reabsorbed (Fig. 5.15b).

During the active phases of the disease the femoral head will assume, due to its plasticity, the shape of the cavity in which it lies. In some instances the femoral head remains within the confines of the acetabulum and as it regenerates is round (Fig. 5.15d). In others antero-lateral subluxation produces an irregular flattened cavity with a corresponding deterioration in head shape (Fig. 5.16c). Metaphyseal changes are commonly extensive. In some cases there is a localised cyst

Fig. 5.14 Group III. Child aged 8 years. No treatment.

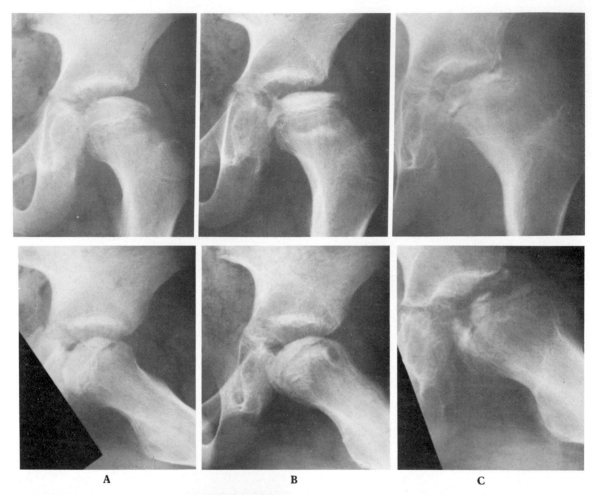

A   B   C

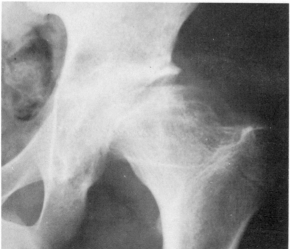

D

Fig. 5.14(a) June 1964. There is a large involved area in the central part of the epiphysis with a good sized medial fragment and a small lateral fragment. There is lateral uncovering of the femoral head, a horizontal growth plate and a diffuse metaphyseal change. The later radiograph shows a small posterior viable fragment and a sclerotic junction between the involved and the uninvolved areas. (**b**) September 1964. There has been further loss of height of the involved segment which is also more dense. The lateral uncovering of the femoral head has become more marked. (**c**) January 1976. Healing is now established but there is considerable head deformity. The metaphyseal lesion has resolved.

Fig. 5.14(d) January 1979. The final result is poor. The sagging rope sign is present.

Fig. 5.15 Group IV. Child aged 2 years. Treatment — Snyder sling.

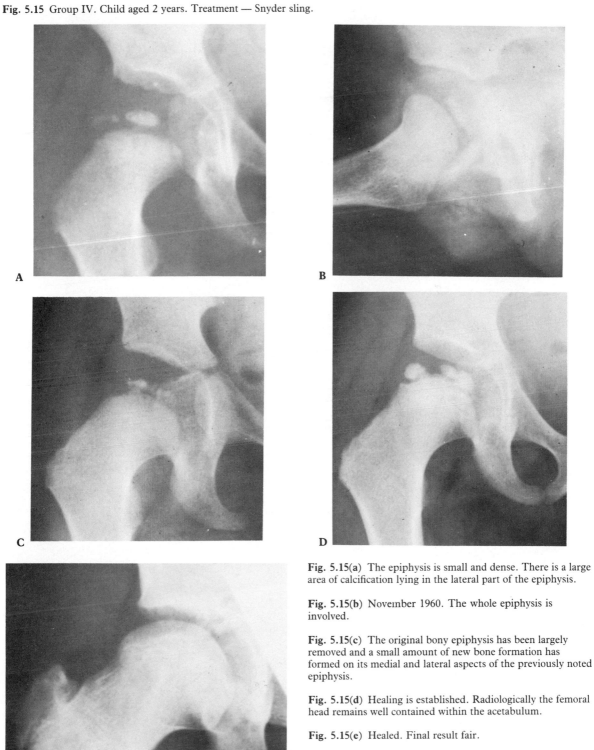

Fig. 5.15(a) The epiphysis is small and dense. There is a large area of calcification lying in the lateral part of the epiphysis.

Fig. 5.15(b) November 1960. The whole epiphysis is involved.

Fig. 5.15(c) The original bony epiphysis has been largely removed and a small amount of new bone formation has formed on its medial and lateral aspects of the previously noted epiphysis.

Fig. 5.15(d) Healing is established. Radiologically the femoral head remains well contained within the acetabulum.

Fig. 5.15(e) Healed. Final result fair.

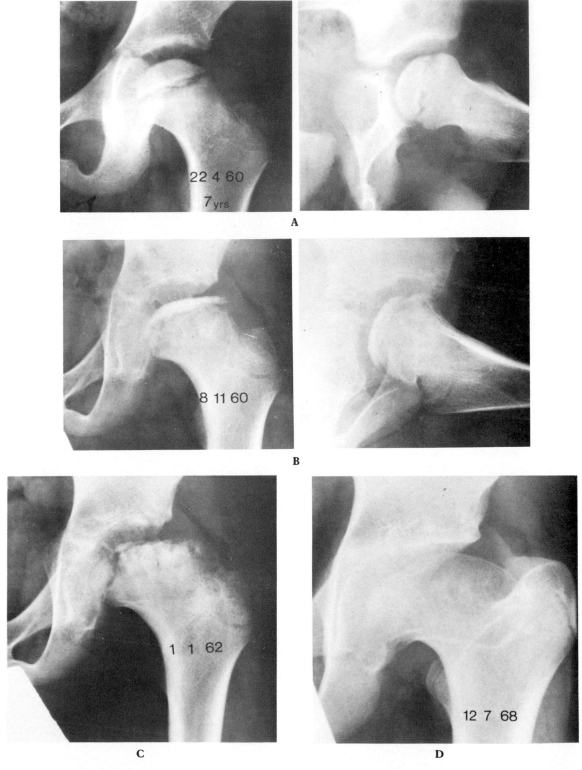

Fig. 5.16 Group IV. Child aged 7 years at diagnosis. Treatment — weight-relieving caliper.

Fig. 5.16(a) April 1960. Antero-posterior radiograph. The epiphysis is generally dense and there is a triangular shape to the medial and lateral aspect of the epiphysis. The lateral radiograph shows that the changes are present throughout the epiphysis and not the anterior part.

Fig. 5.16(b) The antero-posterior radiograph shows total collapse of the epiphysis, widening of the inferomedial joint space and lateral uncovering of the femoral head. The lateral radiograph shows total collapse and remodelling of the posterior metaphysis.

Fig. 5.16(c) January 1962. Healing is now commencing. There is gross flattening and lateral subluxation of the femoral head. **(d)** July 1968. The final result is poor. There has been overgrowth of the greater trochanter.

---

which is usually central on both the antero-posterior and lateral radiographs.

The course of the disease is similar to that in other Groups in that the dense bone must be removed before regeneration can occur. In this Group the duration of the disease is long.

Results in untreated cases

In 1970 I undertook a retrospective review of the notes and radiographs of 388 cases collected from many centres in the British Isles. From these I was able to collect 95 untreated hips. The average follow-up for these cases was 6 years and the male to female ratio 4:1. At the time of final radiograph the result was graded good, fair, or poor according to the following criteria. A good result (Fig. 5.17) was one in which the hip caused no symptoms and had a full range of movement. Radiologically the head was round and well contained within the acetabulum which showed no adaptive changes, the medial joint space was increased. Some loss of epiphyseal height was accepted provided the

femoral head was round. A fair result (Fig. 5.18) was one in which the hip caused no symptoms but movements were a little restricted, especially internal rotation. Radiologically the femoral head was round but a little broadened and might not be fully contained within the acetabulum, up to one fifth being uncovered. Some adaptive changes in the acetabulum were accepted provided the femoral head was round. There was always loss of epiphyseal height. A poor result (Fig. 5.19) was defined as one in which the hip might not be completely symptom free and always showed restriction of movement, especially rotation. Radiologically the head was flattened, broad, irregular, and at least one fifth uncovered. There were adaptive changes in the acetabulum and widening of the inferomedial joint space. This grading is essentially that suggested by Sundt (1949) and it is useful because it reflects the incidence of osteoarthritis in the long term.

Using these criteria the results of untreated cases are shown in Table 5.5. In this you will see that 92 per cent of the good results are seen in Groups I and II and 91 per cent of the poor results in Groups III and IV. Fair results are spread evenly through the Groups.

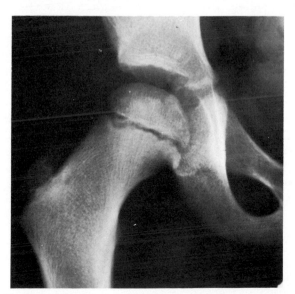

Fig. 5.17 A good result.

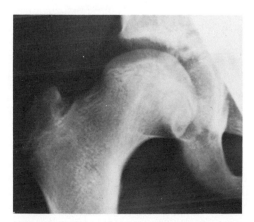

Fig. 5.18 A fair result.

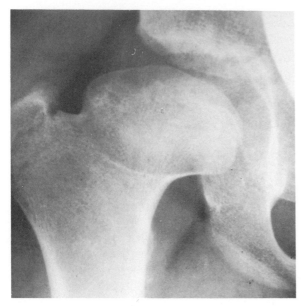

Fig. 5.19 A poor result.

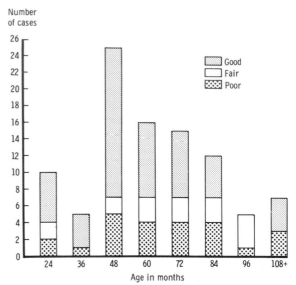

Fig. 5.20 The results in relation to age.

Table 5.5 Results of 95 untreated hips (1970 Survey)

	Good	Fair	Poor
Group I	27	1	0
	92%		
Group II	25	6	2
Group III	4	7	11
			91%
Group IV	0	4	10
Total	54 (57%)	18 (19%)	23 (24%)

It is a conclusion of this evidence that the prognosis in a case of Legg-Calvé-Perthes' disease is proportional to the degree of radiological involvement of the epiphysis. This may be established from a study of the early radiographs and corresponds to the degree of infarction present within the epiphysis. The Groups do not change.

The age and sex ratios within the Groups

Previous reports (Moller 1926, Eyre-Brooke 1936) have suggested that the age of onset and the sex are important in prognosis: the younger boy, particularly, having a more favourable outcome. These factors may be considered in relation to the Groups described.

Age

When the final result is considered in relation to age it is seen that fair and poor results are seen at all ages but that the number of good results becomes substantially reduced over the age of 5 years (Fig. 5.20). It might be suggested that this was because lesser degrees of radiological involvement were seen in younger children. However, when the age of onset is examined within the Groups (Table 5.6), it is noted that although the average age of onset is 72 months this does not differ markedly within the Groups. It is suggested, therefore, that the age of onset is important, firstly because younger children are lighter and therefore less likely to damage their epiphysis and secondly and more importantly because they have longer to remodel their epiphysis after healing of the disease (Fig. 5.21). If it is accepted that Groups II and III cases are a spectrum of disease of common morphology then there is a milder Group II form seen commonly in boys, of shorter duration and occurring at a younger age, whereas in

Table 5.6 Age at presentation within the group (1970 Survey)

	No.	Male:Female Ratio	Average age in months
All Cases	388	3.67:1	72 ± 24.9
Group I	30	14:1	60 ± 18
Group II	143	3.7:1	75 ± 24
Group III	107	2.5:1	80 ± 26
Group IV	43	2.9:1	59 ± 20

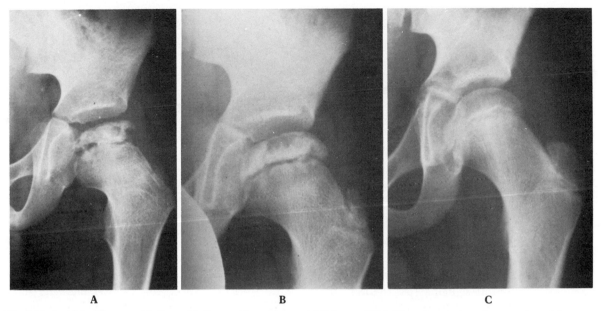

A   B   C

Fig. 5.21 A child of 5 years with Group II disease. No treatment. (a) February 1957. There is some lateral uncovering of the epiphysis. Gage's sign is present. (b) August 1958. At the time of healing the result is fair. (c) January 1967. The final result is good as the result of growth and remodelling.

Table 5.7 Age at presentation in relation to Group and Sex (1970 Survey)

		No.	Average age in months
Boys	Group II	113	74 ± 24
	III	75	83 ± 25
Girls	Group II	30	77 ± 25
	III	32	71 ± 25

Table 5.8 Age at presentation in relation to Group and Sex (1970 Survey)

		No.	Average age in months
Boys	Group I	28	61 ± 18
	IV	32	60 ± 21
Girls	Group I	2	58
	IV	11	55

Group III the reverse is true. There are a greater number of girls in the Group III cases but interestingly their age of onset is similar within Groups II and III cases, and is older than those seen in Groups I and IV (Tables 5.7 and 5.8). There is no obvious explanation for this difference.

Comparison of Groups I and IV cases reveals additional factors of interest (Table 5.8). The age of onset of these two Groups is almost the same and, particularly with the associated high incidence of renal disease, could suggest another subtype in which the Group IV cases were complicated by repeated episodes of infarction. Further evidence, however, will be required to support this data.

Sex

Although the sex ratio overall is 3.67:1 (Table 5.6) it is noted that the ratio for Group I is 14:1 and for

Group IV 2.9:1. This suggests that the poor prognosis for girls is due to the fact that they have a more serious form of the disease. There is no serious difference in outcome between the two sexes within the individual Groups.

Metaphyseal changes

Many workers (Edgren 1965, Ellis 1976, Mindell and Sherman 1951, Langenskiold 1980) have commented on the influence of metaphyseal changes suggesting that the presence of extensive lesions in this area adversely influence the prognosis. It has been noted in the study of the morphology of this condition that two types of changes are observed. Firstly there is widening of the growth plate with islands of cartilage streaming down into the metaphysis and secondly a localised defect usually situated anteriorly and in close relationship to the growth plate. Radiologically two types of lesion

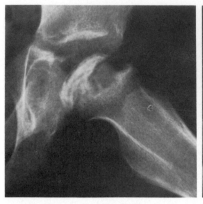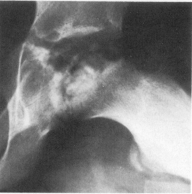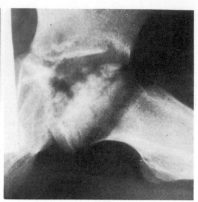

Fig. 5.22 Lateral radiographs of a child with Group III disease showing an extensive metaphyseal lesion. Note that as the disease progresses there is persisting growth of the posterior part of the femoral head and a major alteration in the line of the growth plate as a consequence of the extensive metaphyseal lesion.

may be observed. There is a diffuse area of relative radiolucency stretching across the metaphysis under the involved segment which may be helpful in delineating the extent of the lesion (Fig. 5.22). Secondly there is a localised lytic area which may be small and round or may be extensive involving a large part of the anterior metaphysis (Fig. 5.11a, b). These lesions are well defined with a sclerotic margin on their deep surface and on occasions have no cortical surface on their anterior and lateral margins. They are present during the active phase of the disease only. One of the earliest signs of healing is a progressive reossification of the area producing an apparent alteration in the axis of the growth plate.

It has been noted in the discussion of the morphology that these lesions are associated with a growth disturbance in the femoral neck. It is of interest to note the extent of this abnormality by measuring the ratio of neck length to width in untreated cases, and comparing this with the uninvolved side of unilateral cases (Table 5.9). It will

be observed that there is a steady increase in the ratio with time in the uninvolved hips and those destined for a good result. The poor results showed a reduction in the ratio. This implies broadening of the femoral head with shortening of the femoral neck. Similar changes have been noticed by Robinchon (1974) and shown to follow experimental infarction of the upper femoral epiphysis in animals. In human cases the growth disturbance in the antero-lateral part of the femoral head may explain the increase in femoral antiversion reported by Fabry et al (1973) but does not explain the similar changes on the uninvolved side.

Duration of the disease

It has been the clinical impression of a number of workers in this field that the longer the duration of the disease the worse the long-term result. Lloyd-Roberts et al (1976) have reported that disease of 21 months duration represents a contraindication to operation as it is in this group that the poor results are found.

In the untreated series of cases two interesting factors have been observed. Firstly, the duration of the disease is proportional to the severity of the process, being shorter in Group I than Group IV, not only to the onset of healing but also its overall duration (Table 5.10). It will be seen in the Chapter on Treatment that one of the effects of femoral osteotomy is to initiate an early onset of the healing phase. This may be regarded as one of the im-

Table 5.9 Change in neck ratio with overall result untreated cases

	Uninvolved hips	Good	Fair	Poor
Initial ratio NL/NW	1.66	1.50	1.45	1.42
Final	1.72	1.72	1.47	1.2
Change	+0.06	+0.22	+0.02	−0.22
Number	260	30	22	22

Table 5.10 Duration of disease in relation to group untreated cases

	No.	Healing	Healed
Group I	16	9.0 ± 6.9	24.8 ± 14
Group II	26	9.3 ± 4.4	27.8 ± 9.1
Group III	20	14.6 ± 12 1	31.5 ± 10.1
Group IV	13	17.3 ± 7.2	43.7 ± 13.9

Table 5.11 Duration of disease in relation to results untreated cases

	No.	Healing	Healed
Good	18	11.4 ± 6.5	30.6 ± 8.8
Fair	21	9.5 ± 4.7	31.9 ± 10.9
Poor	14	16 ± 8.6	38.9 ± 12.8

portant effects of femoral osteotomy. Secondly, irrespective of Group the end result is proportional to the duration of disease. It is noted in Table 5.11 that although the time to healing is variable the total duration of the disease is proportional to the result, the good results being on average 8 months shorter than the poor.

The radiological course of the disease and signs of healing

In Groups II, III and IV, once the disease is established part or all of the bony epiphysis becomes crushed. The process of repair removes the crushed avascular bone producing the appearance of fragmentation (Fig. 5.8). This appearance will be accentuated by the presence of small areas of ossification in the thickened articular cartilage, mainly on the lateral aspect of the epiphysis. These areas are initially noted as small areas of ossification (originally considered to be calcification) which gradually enlarge and coalesce. The signs of healing are an increase in the size and height of the medial fragment in Groups II and III cases and an increase in the quality, size and height of the areas of ossification laterally in Groups II, III and IV cases (Fig. 5.8). Once these appearances become established the clinical evidence suggests that no further deterioration will occur in overall head shape (Ferguson and Howarth 1934, Thompson and Westin 1979 and Catterall 1981). This is an important concept as if treatment is to be advised at this time it must be

shown to be effective in containing the femoral head within the mould of the acetabulum.

Healing may be deemed complete when all areas of fibrocartilagenous material within the bony epiphysis have become reossified and there is an increase in the overall height of the central area of the bony epiphysis. At this time the final phase of the disease, namely that of remodelling, commences. Somerville (1971) has noted that provided the femoral head remains contained within the acetabulum this remodelling process will continue until the cessation of growth.

Osteochondritis dissecans

A number of authors have commented on the occurrence of osteochondritis dissecans following Legg-Calvé-Perthes' disease (Guilleminet and Barbier 1957, Freehafer 1960, Morris and McGibbon 1962, Kamhi and MacEwen 1975, Goldman et al 1976 and Hallel and Salvati 1976). The literature contains only 54 reported cases proving the relative rarity of this condition. The site of the osteochondritic fragment is usually in the dome of the healing epiphysis. In the published reports there is no direct correlation between the incidence of this condition and the severity of the disease or the type of treatment utilised. On occasions the lesion may become symptomatic presenting the symptoms of an osteocartilagenous loose body. Goldman et al (1976) states that this occurs approximately 9 years after healing of the disease.

It has been seen in Chapter 4 that during the healing of the disease process clefts may be seen in the fibrocartilagenous material in the dome of the epiphysis. If ossification occurred in the cartilage overlying such a cleft by the invasion of the vascular granulation tissue from its periphery, then an area of osteochondritis would form. A second mechanism may, however, also occur. In any Group where there is fibrocartilagenous material in the superior part of the epiphysis, ossification occurs following the invasion of granulation tissue through the sides of the defect and through its deep margin. Should these areas of ossification fail to coalesce then an area of osteochondritis may form. This latter process may be considered as similar to hypertrophic nonunion of a fracture; the movement of the fragment occurring as the result

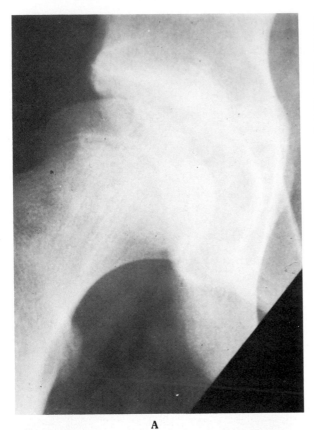

A

Fig. 5.23 A child aged 12 years with healed Group III disease. He presented with acute episodes of pain. On two occasions the joint has become stuck.

Fig. 5.23(a) The plain radiograph shows healed Perthes' disease.

Fig. 5.23(b) The arthrogram wiith a large osteochondritic fragment situated in the superior aspect of the joint having eroded a defect in the roof of the acetabulum.

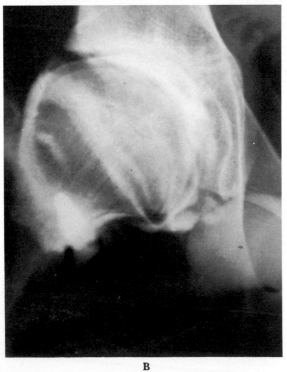

B

B

of normal activities such as walking and running.

Unless the fragment becomes loose as reported by Goldman et al (1976) the joint remains totally without symptoms (Ratliff 1967). In a personal case (Fig. 5.23) the osteochondritic fragment was difficult to observe on the plain films although the clinical symptoms were those of recurrent episodes of sharp mechanical pain. The diagnosis was only established by arthrography which is therefore indicated in any cases in which symptoms of a mechanical nature occur during the healing and remodelling phases of the disease process.

REFERENCES

Anderson J, Stewart A M 1970 The significance of the magnitude of the medial hip space. British Journal of Radiology 43: 238–239

Blakemore M E, Harrison M H M 1979 A prospective study of children with untreated Catterall Group I Perthes' disease. Journal of Bone and Joint Surgery 61B: 329–333

Bobechko W, Harris W R 1960 Radiographic density of avascular bone Journal of Bone and Joint Surgery 42B: 626–632

Burrows H J, 1941 Coxa plana with special reference to its pathology and kinship. British Journal of Surgery 29: 23–36

Burrows H J 1954 Annotation osteochondritis juvenilis. Journal of Bone and Joint Surgery 41B: 455–456

Caffey J 1968 The early roentgenographic changes in essential coxa vara: significance in pathogenesis. American Journal of Roentgenology 103: 620–634

Calvé J 1910 Sur une forme particulare de pseudo-coxalgia greffe sur des deformations caracteristiques de l'extremite superiure due femur. Revue de Chirurgie 30: 54–84

Catterall A 1970 Personal observations.

Catterall A 1971 The natural history of Perthes's disease. Journal of Bone and Joint Surgery 53B: 37–53

Catterall A 1981 Legg-Calvé-Perthes' syndrome. Clinical Orthopaedics and Related Research. 158: 41–52

Crossan J F 1980 Personal communications

Dolman C L, Bell H M 1973 The pathology of Legg-Calvé-Perthes' disease. Journal of Bone and Joint Surgery 55A: 184–188

Edgren W 1965 Coxa Plana. A clinical and radiological investigation with particular reference to the importance of the metaphyseal changes for the final shape of the proximal part of the femur. Acta Orthopaedica Scandinavica Suppl. 84

Ellis W 1976 The metaphysis in Perthes' disease: a method of assessment and selection for weight bearing. Journal of Bone and Joint Surgery 58B: 368–369

Eyre-Brooke A L 1936 Osteochondritis deformans coxae juvenilis or Perthes' disease. The results of treatment by traction in recumbancy. British Journal of Surgery 24: 166–182

Fabrey G, MacEwen G D, Shands A R 1973 Torsion of the femur. Journal of Bone and Joint Surgery 55A: 1726

Ferguson A B 1954 Synovitis of the hip and Legg-Calvé-Perthes' disease — observations on the outline of the capsule shadow. Clinical Orthopaedics and Related Research 4: 180

Ferguson A B, Howarth M B 1934 A study of coxa plana and related conditions of the hip. Journal of Bone and Joint Surgery 16: 781

Freehafer A A 1960 Osteochondritis dissecans following Legg-Calvé-Perthes' disease Journal of Bone and Joint Surgery 42A: 777–782

Goldman AB, Hallel, T, Salvati E, Freiberger R H 1976 Osteochondritis dessicans complicating Legg-Perthes' disease. Radiology 121: 561–566

Guilleminet M, Barbier J M 1957 Osteochondritis dissecans of the hip. Journal of Bone and Joint Surgery 39B: 268–277

Hallel T, Salvati E A 1976 Osteochondritis dissecans following Legg-Calvé-Perthes' disease. Journal of Bone and Joint Surgery 58A: 708–711

Herring J A, Lundeen M A, Wenger D R 1980 Minimal Perthes' disease Journal of Bone and Joint Surgery 62B: 25–30

Jacobs P 1976 Aseptic Necrosis of Bone. J K Davidson. Excerpta Medica, Amsterdam.

Jansen M 1923 On coxa plana and its causation. Journal of Bone and Joint Surgery 5: 265–277

Jonaster S 1953 Coxa plana — a histo-pathological and arthrographic study. Acta Orthopaedica Scandinavica Suppl. 12

Kamhi E, MacEwen G D 1975 Osteochondritis dissecans in Legg-Calvé-Perthes' disease. Journal of Bone and Joint Surgery 57A: 506

Kemp H B S, Boldero J L 1966 Radiological changes in Perthes' disease British Journal of Radiology 39: 744–760

Langenskiold A L 1980 Changes in the capital growth plate and the proximal femoral metaphysis in Legg-Calvé-Perthes' disease. Clinical Orthopaedics and Related Research 150: 110–114

Legg A T 1910 An obscure affection of the hip joint. Boston Medical and Surgical Journal 162: 202–204

Lloyd-Roberts G C, Catterall A, Salamon P B 1976 A controlled study of the indications and results of femoral osteotomy in Perthes' disease. Journal of Bone and Joint Surgery 58B: 31–36

Mindell E R, Sherman M S 1951 Late results in Legg-Perthes' disease. Journal of Bone and Joint Surgery 33A 1–23

Moller P F 1926 Clinical observations after healing of Calvé-Perthes' disease compared with the final deformities on the ultimate prognosis. Acta Radiologica 5:1

Morris M L, McGibbon K C 1962 Osteochondritis dissecans following Legg-Calvé-Perthes' disease. Journal of Bone and Joint Surgery 44B: 562–564

O'Garra J A 1959 The radiographic changes in Perthes' disease. Journal of Bone and Joint Surgery 41B: 465–476

Perthes G C 1910 Uber arthritis deformans juvenilis. Deutsche Zeitschrift fur Chirurgie. 107: 11–59

Ralston E L 1961 Legg-Calvé-Perthes' disease — factors in healing Journal of Bone and Joint Surgery 43A 249–260

Ratcliff A H C 1967b Osteochondritis dissecans following Legg-Calvé-Perthes' disease. Journal of Bone and Joint Surgery 49B: 108–111

Robichon J, Desjardins J P, Koch M, Hooper C E, 1974 The femoral neck in Legg-Perthes' disease — its relationship to epiphyseal change and its importance in early prognosis. Journal of Bone and Joint Surgery 56B 62–68

Salter R B, Thompson G H 1980 Legg-Calvé-Perthes' disease. The prognostic significance of the subchondral fracture. Paper presented to the American Academy of Orthopaedic Surgeons 1980

Somerville E W 1971 Perthes' disease of the hip. Journal of Bone and Joint Surgery 53B: 639–649

Sundt H 1949 Further investigations respecting mature Coxae-Calvé-Legg-Perthes' disease with special regard to prognosis and treatment. Acta Chirugica Scandinavica Suppl. 148

Thompson G H, Westin G W 1979 Legg-Clavé Perthes' disease — results of discontinuing treatment in the early re-ossification phase. Clinical Orthopaedics and Related Research 139: 70–80

Waldenström H 1909 Der obere tuberkulose collumherd. Zeitschrift fur Orthopadische Chirurgie. 24: 487–512

Waldenström H 1920 Coxa plana, osteochondritis deformans coxae, Calvé-Perthessche Krankheit, Legg disease. Zentralblatt fur Chirurgie 47: 539–542

Waldenström H 1923 On coxa plana, osteochondritis deformans coxae juvenilis. Leggs disease, Maladie de Calvé, Perthes Krankheit. Acta Chirugica Scandinavica 55: 577–590

Waldenström H 1934 The first stage of coxa plana. Acta Orthopaedica Scandinavica 5: 1–34

Waldenström H 1938 The first stages of coxa plana. Journal of Bone and Joint Surgery 20: 559–566

6

The long term prognosis

Historical review

It is in the anticipation of the high incidence of osteoarthritis (Fig. 6.1) which many cases of Legg-Calvé-Perthes' disease will develop in the long term, that the controversies on treatment really arise. It should be the aim of treatment to prevent these changes. The literature on the long term consequences is fortunately small and relatively uniform in its conclusions (Moller 1924, Sundt 1949, Helbo 1953, Evans 1958, Danielsson 1964, 1965, Ratcliff 1956, 1967, 1977, Eaton 1967, Gower and Johnston 1971, Steinhauser 1971, Brotherton and McKibbin 1977, Meyer 1977, Mose et al 1977, and Hall 1980). The general conclusion is that in the long term, despite the high incidence of radiological osteoarthritis, the symptoms attributable to it are often long delayed (Fig. 6.2). At 40 years Ratcliff (1977) has shown that one third of cases have a good, fair or poor result. Brotherton and McKibbin (1977) are the only authors to comment on the high incidence of successful asymptomatic results following a period of treatment by containment in wide abduction in which weight-bearing was not permitted. The most complete and authoritative of the long term follow-up accounts is that of Mose et al (1977) who have reviewed the long term results of three series reported initially by Moller (1924), Helbo (1953) and Mose (1964). Their conclusions are that, although 86 per cent of cases may be expected to develop the symptoms of osteoarthritis by the age of 65 years, between the ages of 25 and 35 years there is a relatively low incidence (6 per cent) of severe radiological or clinical signs. The subsequent onset of osteoarthritis is proportional to the shape of the head, both at

presentation and at the time of healing. The irregular uncovered femoral head has the greatest incidence of osteoarthritis, becomes stiffer at an earlier stage, and has a higher incidence of severe pain than other types of femoral head shape. There is a strong correlation between the age of onset of the disease and the incidence of arthritis; younger children having statistically lower incidence of arthritis compared with disease starting over the age of 9 years. Hall (1980) has recently reviewed 103 cases with an average follow-up of 32 years. In general he has confirmed the findings of Mose et al (1977) but has been concerned mainly with prognostic factors. He has shown that in the long term there is no correlation with sphericity (Mose radius), epiphyseal quotient, C.E. angle, or visual assessments taken at the time of healing. The only useful factor relating to long term prognosis was the head-height measurement (E.A.) at this stage. This sign was initially described by Catterall (1971) as a sign of value in the interpretation of arthrographic appearances.

The 1970 review

There were 75 cases in which there was a 10 year follow-up or more and from a study of these cases a number of factors were found to be of importance. These are the age of the patient at the time of healing, persistent lateral uncovering, the presence of a premature growth plate arrest and severe flattening of the femoral head (Table 6.1)

Age at the time of healing

Although many authors have commented on the

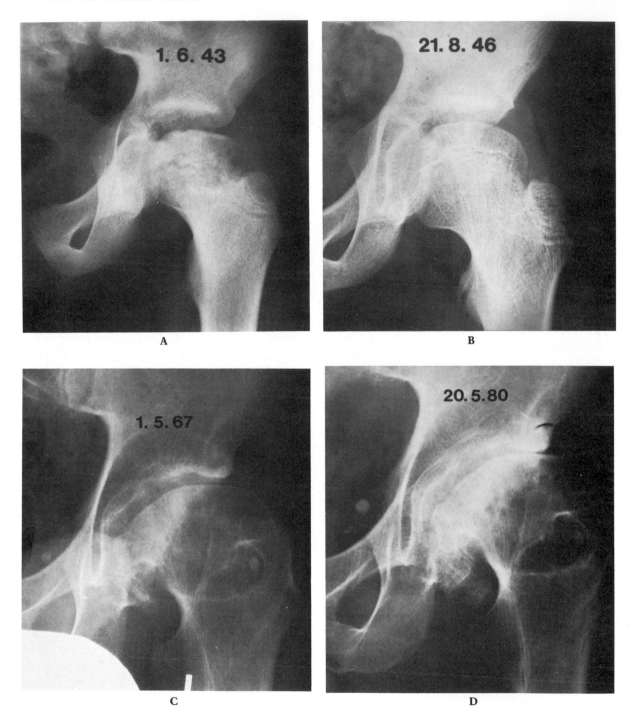

Fig. 6.1(a) June 1943. A child aged 5 years 6 months with established Group II disease.

Fig. 6.1(b) August 1946. Treatment by bed rest has resulted in a fair result.

Fig. 6.1(c) May 1967. He presented with mild hip symptoms responding to conservative treatment. The sagging rope sign is present.

Fig. 6.1(d) May 1980. He is now getting regular hip symptoms including limitation of activity and occasional pain at night.

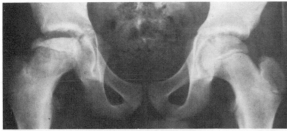

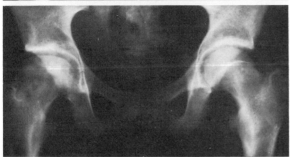

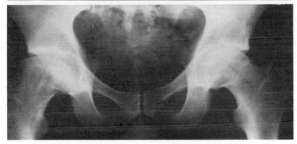

Fig. 6.2(**a**, top) May 1947. A child aged 7 years with Group III disease involving the right hip. (**b**, middle) May 1950. Following 1 year of bed rest and 1 year in a weight-relieving caliper healing is complete. There is femoral head deformity but a well preserved joint space superiorly and medially. (**c**, bottom) August 1967. Left hip remains asymptomatic with good preservation of joint space, early osteophyte formation and a sagging rope sign is noted on the right side.

Table 6.1 Factors influencing long term prognosis (1970 Survey)

---

1. Age at the time of healing
2. Severe flattening of the femoral head
3. Persistent lateral uncovering
4. Premature arrest of the growth plate.

Table 6.2 Changes in result in the long term (1970 Survey)

75 Cases	— 25 improved	— 20 one result category
		— 5 two result categories
	— 11 deteriorated	

age of the patient at diagnosis (Moller 1926, Eyre-Brooke 1936), few have commented on the importance of age at the time of healing. Both Snyder (1975) and Clarke et al (1978) have emphasised that a proportion of patients who have an early onset of the disease achieve a poor result although in general younger children fair better in the long term than older ones. I have confirmed that in general younger children do have a better prognosis but that poor results may be seen in disease starting even at the age of 2 years. The reason for this is not that they have a milder form of the disease, but because they have longer to remodel their femoral head after healing is established. It must be remembered that remodelling cannot commence until healing is established. In the older child, particularly with Groups III or IV disease, this factor would seem to be of importance especially where any form of treatment is able to initiate the healing process.

In this series there were 75 cases with a minimum follow-up of 10 years or more. Of these 25 or one third had improved by one or more result categories and of these 5 had improved by two result categories (Table 6.2). In these latter 5 cases the disease had started under the age of 5 years. More interestingly 11 cases had deteriorated. The common features in this deterioration were the irregular shaped femoral head at the time of healing, the presence of a premature growth arrest of part or all of the growth plate and persistent lateral uncovering.

Severe flattening of the femoral head

The poor prognosis in the long term for the femoral head which at the time of healing is irregular and flattened has been confirmed. As will be seen when the problems of treatment are discussed this leads to the phenomenon of Hinge Abduction, resulting in subluxation and an early onset of degenerative change.

Persistent lateral uncovering

The present study has confirmed the fact that uncovering of the femoral head outside the confines of the acetabulum adversely affects the long term prognosis. It is usually considered that this uncovering is the consequence of enlargement of the femoral head laterally. Little attention has been paid to the thought that part of this uncovering could be due to a failure of the lateral lip of the acetabulum to maintain adequate growth. It is remarkable to see in the younger child how overgrowth of the acetabular side of the hip joint allows satisfactory long term remodelling despite broadening of the femoral head. This growth potential will be considered in detail when the 'potential for remaining growth' is discussed (p. 86). It should be stated, however, that where the phenomenon of Hinge Abduction persists there is mechanical deformation of the lateral fibrocartilagenous portion of the acetabulum and a failure of normal lateral growth. This can be remedied by correcting the phenomenon of hinging, by abduction osteotomy (Fig. 8.20).

Premature arrest of the growth plate

A number of authors have commented on the adverse effect on the long term prognosis of premature closure of the growth plate, Ratcliff (1956), Langenskiold and Salenius (1967), Schiller and Axer (1972), Edgren (1975), Kamhi and MacEwen (1975) and Barnes (1980). Synder (1975) considered that this is the main cause of the poor result in the younger child. This poor prognosis has been confirmed in the present study and it is considered that premature growth plate arrest interferes with the long term remodelling process. Radiologically two types of change may be observed, a partial or complete closure. In the complete type (Fig. 6.3) a complete arrest of the whole growth plate occurs. This results in a short neck, often with a high greater trochanter but with a normal shaped femoral head often well seated within the acetabulum. In the partial type (Fig. 6.4) two appearances are recognised. There is, firstly, a bridge of bone which forms usually at the lateral margin of the original growth plate, resulting in a cessation of growth in this area and persisting growth laterally. Secondly, there is the disorganisation of the anterior and lateral part of the growth plate which occurs as a consequence of the extensive metaphyseal lesion which even when healed has a disorganised structure and therefore abnormal growth.

Barnes (1980) in a study of problems of premature growth plate arrest has shown that they are most commonly seen in Groups III and IV disease. When surgical treatment has been advised they are particularly prone to occur when treatment has been undertaken during the healing phases of the disease. This adds support to the principle that treatment undertaken at this time must be shown to improve effectively containment of the femoral head. Failure to follow this principle may result in premature growth arrest which may actually reverse the good effects of treatment.

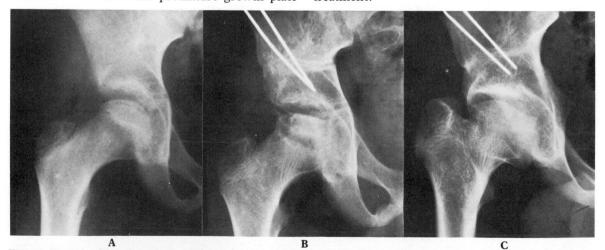

Fig. 6.3 Example of complete arrest of the growth plate. (a) February 1974. A child with Group III disease aged 9 years. (b) September 1974. After initial mobilisation an innominate osteotomy was performed. The femoral head is well contained but an extensive metaphyseal lesion is noted. (c) March 1976. The head is remaining round and well contained within the acetabulum. There has been a complete arrest of the growth plate resulting in a short neck and an elevated greater trochanter.

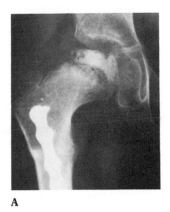

A

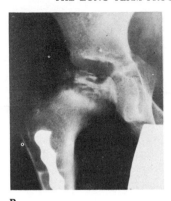

B

Fig. 6.4 An example of a partial arrest of the growth plate. (a) January 1975. A Group III disease treated by femoral ostcotomy. (b) December 1974. Healing is well established and an area of endochondral ossification has formed laterally.

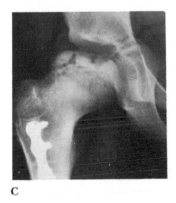

C

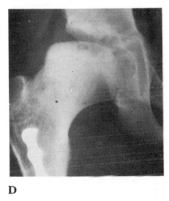

D

Fig. 6.4(c) December 1975. The central area of the epiphysis appears fused but is open on the medial and lateral sides. There is enlargement of the lateral aspect of the head. (**d**) June 1980. The final result, the degree of uncovering has increased as the disease has healed.

Radiological changes in the long term

The most obvious changes observed radiologically in the course of long term follow-up are those of degenerative arthritis (Fig. 6.1). Although in the majority of cases these are confined to the involved head, this is not true in every case. Provided, as the result of healing and long term remodelling, a congruence is achieved between the shape of the femoral head and acetabulum it is remarkable how long the onset of radiological arthritis may be delayed. In these circumstances degenerative changes may involve the opposite uninvolved hip first (Fig. 6.2). This leads to the concept of 'congruous incongruity' as an important long term objective of treatment, a term first used by Burr Curtis.

The sagging rope sign

In some cases of secondary osteoarthritis of the hip joint, there is doubt at the time of presentation of its initial aetiology. A radiological sign called the 'sagging rope sign', originally noted by Perkins and commented on by Evans (1958), and fully described by Appley and Wientroub (1981) is of value in this context (Fig. 6.1c, d, 6.2c). In some cases of osteoarthritis on the antero-posterior radiographs there is a sclerotic line situated in the middle zone of the femoral neck often with an area of osteoporosis above it. There is dispute as to the cause of this radiological appearance. My investigation suggests that this line represents the anterior margin of the femoral head as it angulates acutely to join the metaphyseal area, the cortical bone at this point being seen as a dense line on the antero-posterior view. It is seen in any case where there has been a growth disturbance in the anterior part of the femoral head following avascular necrosis, for example, Legg-Calvé-Perthes' disease, congenital dislocation of the hip and systemic disorders such as multiple epiphyseal dysplasia.

Conclusions

Bearing in mind the relatively good results of this condition in the long term and the degree of femoral head deformity which may be tolerated without the appearance of serious symptoms it is possible to provide indications for treatment during the active phase of the disease. Treatment would be indicated in the older child and in cases in which there is a serious risk of deformity of the femoral head with persistent lateral uncovering. It would be considered effective if it could biologically initiate the healing process without injury to the growth plate.

REFERENCES

Appley A G, Wientroub S 1981 The Sagging Rope Sign in Perthes' disease Journal of Bone and Joint Surgery 63B:

Barnes J M 1980 Premature epiphysial closure in Perthes' disease Journal of Bone and Joint Surgery 62B: 432–437

Brotherton B J, McKibbin B 1977 Perthes' disease treated by prolonged rucumbancy and femoral head containment, a long term appraisal Journal of Bone and Joint Surgery 59B: 14

Catterall A 1971 The natural history of Perthes' disease. Journal of Bone and Joint Surgery 53B: 37–53

Clarke T E, Finnegan T L, Fisher R L, Bunch W H, Gossling H R 1978 Legg-Perthes' disease in children less than four years old Journal of Bone and Joint Surgery 60A: 166

Curtis B H 1978 Personal communication

Danielsson L G 1964 Incidence and prognosis of coxarthrosis Acta Orthopaedica Scandinavica suppl. 66: 14–20

Danielsson L G Late result of Perthes' disease. Acta Orthopaedica Scandinavica 36: 70–81

Eaton G O 1967 Long term results of treatment in coxa plana. Journal of Bone and Joint Surgery 49A: 1031–1042

Edgren W 1965 Coxa plana. A clinical and radiological investigation with particular reference to the importance of the metaphyseal changes for the final shape of the proximal part of the femur. Acta Orthopaedica Scandinavica Spuul. 84

Evans D L 1958 Legg-Calvé-Perthes' disease. A study of late results. Journal of Bone and Joint Surgery 40B: 168–181

Eyre-Brooke A L 1936 Osteochondritis deformans coxae juvenilis or Perthes' disease. The results of treatment by traction in recumbancy. British Journal of Surgery 24: 166–182

Gower W E, Johnson R C 1971 Legg-Perthes' disease, long term follow-up of thirty-six patients. Journal of Bone and Joint Surgery 53A: 759–768

Hall G 1980 Some observations on Perthes' disease. Robert Jones Prize Essay of the British Orthopaedica Association

Helbo S 1953 Morbus Calvé-Perthes. Thesis, Copenhagen, Fyns Tidendes Bogtrykkeri, Odense.

Kamhi E, MacEwen G D 1975 Osteochondritis dissecans in Legg-Calve-Perthes' disease. Journal of Bone and Joint Surgery 57A: 506

Langenskiold A, Salenius P 1967 Epiphyseodesis of the greater trochanter Acta Orthopaedica Scandinavica 38: 199

Meyer J 1977 Legg-Calvé-Perthes' disease, radiological results of treatment and their late consequences. Acta Orthopaedica Scandinavica Suppl. 167

Moller P E 1924 Malum deformans coxae infantile. Thesis, Kohenhayn.

Moller P F 1926 Clinical observations after healing of Calve-Perthes' disease compared with the final deformities left by that disease, and bearing of those final deformites on the ultimate prognosis. Acta Radiological 5: 1

Mose K 1964 Legg-Calvé-Perthes' disease, results of treatment. A comparison between three methods of conservative treatment. Copenhagen Universitetsforlaget 1964

Mose K, Hjorth L, Ulfeldt M, Christensen E R, Jensen A 1977 Legg-Calvé-Perthes' disease, the late occurrence of coxarthrosis. Acta Orthopaedica Scandinavica Suppl. 169

Ratcliff A H C 1956 Pseudocoxalgia — a study of late results in the adult. Journal of Bone and Joint Surgery 38B: 498–512

Ratcliff A H C 1967 Perthes' disease. A study of 34 hips observed for 30 years. Journal of Bone and Joint Surgery 49B: 102

Ratcliff A H C 1977 Perthes' disease — a study of 16 patients followed up for 40 years. Journal of Bone and Joint Surgery 59B: 248

Schiller M G, Axer A 1972 Hypertrophy of the femoral head ir Legg-Calvé-Perthes' syndrome. Acta Orthopaedica Scandinavica 43: 45–55

Snyder C R 1975 Legg-Calvé-Perthes' disease in the young hip — does it necessarily do well? Journal of Bone and Joint Surgery 57A: 751–758

Steinhauser E 1971 Spatergebnisse der perthesschen Krankheit. Zeitschrift Orthopaedica 107: 558–576

Sundt H 1949 Further investigations respecting mature coxae-Calve-Legg-Perthes' disease with special regard to prognosis and treatment. Acta Chirugica Scandinavica Suppl. 148

7

The poor result

It follows from the discussion of the radiological features and the long term prognosis that with a condition in which nearly 60 per cent do well without treatment, great attention should be focussed on those cases destined for a poor result. Where possible these poor results should be diagnosed early during the active phase of the disease and appropriate treatment started. It must, however, be stressed that overall deterioration in the shape of the femoral head can occur not only during the active phase of the disease but also in the remodelling period, if there is any failure of the normal growth in part or all of the growth plate. The early diagnosis of those cases in which severe flattening of the femoral head is going to occur can only be made with the knowledge of the mechanism of femoral head deformity and of the radiological signs associated with this change.

The mechanism of femoral head deformity

It has been seen, when the morphological changes were discussed, that in Groups II, III and IV cases there is an increasing degree of infarction in the epiphysis. Associated with this there is an overgrowth of the articular cartilage. This is proportional to the degree of ischaemia and is most marked in the Group IV cases. Associated with these two processes part or all of the bony epiphysis may become crushed. Following this infarction a process of repair lays appositional new bone on the surface of intact trabeculae. Those trabeculae which are crushed become progressively reabsorbed from their deep margin, and replaced by a fibrocartilagenous material in which ossification slowly occurs. During the healing phase of the disease the thickened articular cartilage is ossified by endochondral ossification seen particularly in the anterior and lateral aspects of the deformed femoral head. The thick fibrocartilagenous material is gradually reossified from its deep surface. This will produce different rates of growth in various parts of the femoral head and therefore deformity.

Clinically it is observed that the femoral head in which deformity is occurring lies adducted and has a reduced range of movement. This is the consequence of four processes. Firstly, there is enlargement of the cartilagenous portion of the femoral head as the result of continuing growth of the cartilage following infarction of the epiphysis and also in some cases as the result of a primary abnormality occurring before the disease becomes active. Secondly, there is crushing of part or all of the bony epiphysis. Thirdly, these two factors together produce an upward and lateral displacement of the femoral head which is in part a true subluxation and in part a growth disturbance. Radiologically this is observed as a break in Shenton's line (Fig. 7.1). Fourthly, the femoral head comes to lie in an adducted position which is then maintained by adductor spasm finally producing an adduction contracture (Table 7.1).

Once the adducted position has been reached the growth disturbance which has already been discussed produces an overgrowth of the medial

Table 7.1 Causes of adduction deformity

1. Overgrowth of articular cartilage particularly on the medical and lateral aspect of the femoral head.

2. Crushing of the trabeculae within the epiphysis

Producing:

3. Upward and lateral displacement of the femoral head

4. Adductor spasm leading to adduction contracture

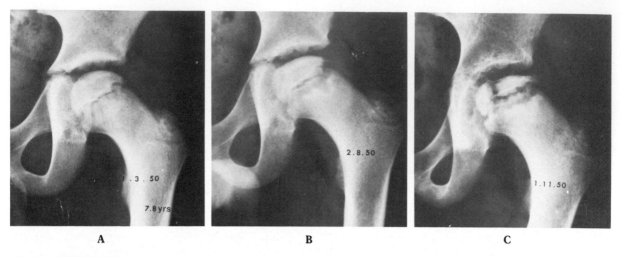

| A | B | C |

Fig. 7.1(a) March 1950. Boy aged 7 years 8 months with early disease. A subchondral fracture line can be seen extending across the dome of the femoral head suggesting Group III disease. No at-risk signs. (**b**) August 1950. There is resorption of the lateral part of the femoral epiphysis (Gage's sign) with lateral calcification and a diffuse metaphyseal change. There is an early break in Shenton's line with loss of height of the epiphysis and widening of the inferomedial joint space. These are signs of the head-at-risk. (**c**) November 1950. Marked break in Shenton's line with uncovering of the lateral aspect the femoral head and further loss of epiphyseal height.

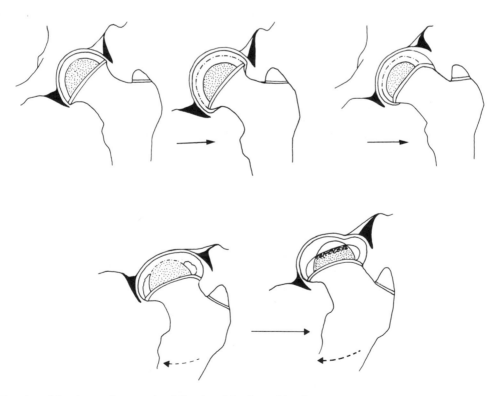

Fig. 7.2 Drawing of the phases of progressive deformity of the femoral head.

and lateral aspects of the femoral head, thereby contributing to the deformity (Fig. 7.2). This is best recognised by an examination of hips obtained at necropsy where it is seen that the dent in the anterior and lateral aspect of the femoral head corresponds to the weight-bearing position of the femoral head if the hip lies in the flexed and adducted position (Fig. 3.11f).

Once this degree of femoral head deformity has occurred the normal movement of the hip becomes altered. In the normal child the movements of abduction and flexion are pure rotation, whereas when femoral head deformity is present the movement is initially one of rotation with hinging (Fig. 7.3). With progressive deformity and uncovering of the femoral head lateral to the bony acetabulum the process of abduction changes to one of pure hinging, a phenomenon called 'hinge abduction'. This produces a dent in the lateral part of the femoral head (Fig. 7.4). In these cir-

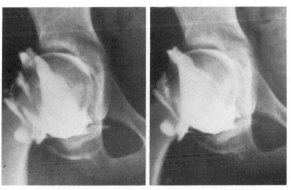

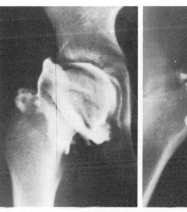

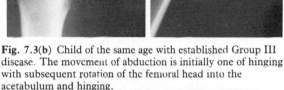

Fig. 7.3(a) Arthrogram of child aged 5 years with a normal head on the left in the neutral position and on the right in abduction. The movement is one of pure rotation.

Fig. 7.3(b) Child of the same age with established Group III disease. The movement of abduction is initially one of hinging with subsequent rotation of the femoral head into the acetabulum and hinging.

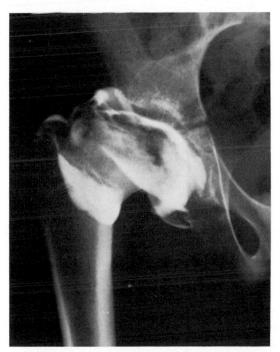

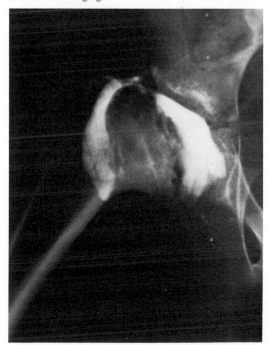

Fig. 7.4 Arthrogram of child with major deformity of the femoral head showing the phenomenon of hinge abduction.

cumstances the subluxation becomes fixed and the processes of differential growth, particularly in the lateral part of the femoral head, contribute to the final deformity. (Fig. 3.11f).

While these changes are occurring in the epiphysis and articular cartilage further changes are observed in the growth plate and metaphysis. It has already been noted that the growth plate is abnormal and therefore a disturbance of normal growth of the femoral neck might be expected. The metaphyseal lesions are areas of unossified cartilage whose cells are capable of proliferation. Where these areas are in contact with the growth plate the architecture of the plate is lost (Fig. 3.11k). This will result in a loss of longitudinal growth, either locally or generally, in the anterior and lateral part of the femoral neck. This will lead to differential rates of growth within the femoral neck, the magnitude of which will be proportional to the extent of the metaphyseal lesion.

The result of this growth disturbance in both epiphysis and metaphysis leaves a normal area of growth in the posterior and medial part of the femoral head with progressive tilting of the growth plate due to a growth disturbance of cartilage and growth plate in the antero-lateral part (Fig. 5.22). Crushing of the bony epiphysis exacerbates this deformity. In these circumstances the deformity of the femoral head seems to hinge on the height of the posterior and medial viable fragment with progressive failure of the anterior and lateral aspects of the femoral head to grow at the same rate as the postero-medial part.

Radiological signs of deterioration in the shape of the femoral head

When plain radiographs are reviewed changes in femoral head shape may be considered from three aspects. These are epiphyseal changes, metaphyseal changes, and the presence of lateral subluxation.

Epiphyseal changes

Three types of epiphyseal change may be observed (Table 7.2). These are broadening of the epiphysis, areas of calcification or ossification occurring just lateral to the epiphysis and defects in the lateral

Table 7.2. Radiological signs associated with change in femoral head shape.

Epiphyseal changes	1. Broadening of the epiphysis
	2. Calcification lateral to the epiphysis
	3. Gage's sign
Metaphyseal changes	1. Localised anterior
	2. Diffuse
Lateral subluxation	1. Lateral uncovering

part of the epiphysis and adjacent metaphysis (Gage's sign).

Broadening of the epiphysis. It has already been observed that broadening of the femoral head occurs as the result of ossification in the performed cartilagenous model. This enlargement is in an antero-lateral direction and is in part down the lateral side of the femoral neck. When ossification occurs in this preformed mass of cartilage the shape of the femoral head radiologically changes as does the shape of the lateral part of the growth plate. Apparent flattening of the epiphysis will occur in these circumstances, not simply as the result of loss of height but as a consequence of increased breadth of the femoral head without an associated increase in height (Fig. 7.1c and Fig. 7.2).

Calcification lateral to the epiphysis. This sign was first noticed in association with the Group III cases and is always an important radiological sign. The areas of calcification may be either large (Fig. 7.5) or small (Fig. 7.6. and Fig. 7.1b). These are small islands of ossification lying in the enlarged cartilagenous model. This sign can only be present when enlargement of the femoral head has in fact already occurred. This part of the femoral head, being cartilage, is still plastic as there is no major mass of ossification giving rigidity to it, preventing biological remodelling of the cartilage from occurring. As the mass of calcification or ossification increases, and particularly as it coalesces, the shape of the head becomes less plastic and therefore less amenable to alteration by containment treatment.

Gage's sign. Courtnay Gage (1932) originally described a curved defective area of ossification in the lateral epiphysis and adjacent metaphysis as an early sign of Perthes' disease. This important sign, which is often overlooked, is the consequence of a

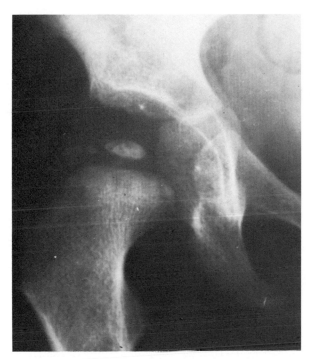

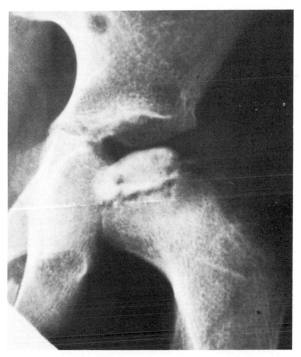

Fig. 7.5 Calcification lateral to the epiphysis. A child aged 2 years 6 months with Group IV disease. There is a large area of calcification/ossification lateral to the involved segment.

Fig. 7.6 Calcification lateral to the epiphysis. Child aged 5 years with Group III disease showing a small area of calcification/ossification lateral to the involved segment.

failure of normal ossification of the cartilage on the lateral aspect of the epiphysis and adjacent metaphysis. In established disease however a similar but different sign is also observed. This may arise as the result of two possible processes. Firstly, there may be reabsorption of the lateral portion of the bony epiphysis leading to a defect in this area (Fig. 7.1b). In other circumstances ossification occurring in the enlarged lateral cartilage mass is in direct continuity with the epiphysis but just above the growth plate producing an apparent lytic area in this region (Fig. 7.7). In either event the radiological signs suggest that there is a mass of articular cartilage lying lateral to the epiphysis and often unconstrained within the mould of the acetabulum. This is therefore a sign suggesting that femoral head deterioration is already present but without major reossification of the deformed segment.

Metaphyseal changes. Radiologically two types of metaphyseal lesion are observed. These are localised or diffuse. The localised lesion is usually situated in the anterior and lateral part of the metaphy-

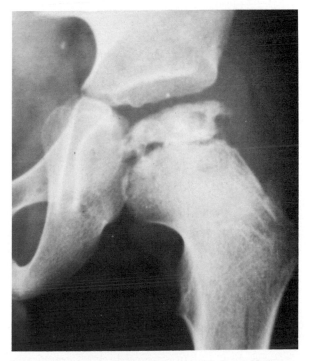

Fig. 7.7 Gage's sign. Child aged 5 years with Group II disease and a defect in the lateral aspect of the epiphysis.

sis under the involved segment, except in the Group IV cases where it may be central in both views. This lesion has a well defined sclerotic margin and reossifies once the healing process is established. The diffuse lesion again lies under the involved segment but its edges are often not so clearly defined, looking more like a generalised thickening of the growth plate itself with irregular ossification on its deep margin. The importance of the growth disturbance associated with these lesions has already been discussed.

Lateral subluxation. In addition to these radiological signs lateral subluxation first noted by Waldenström (1934) is an important sign of impending deterioration of the femoral head. It has been noted that apparent subluxation or uncovering is in many cases a manifestation of a growth disturbance with enlargement of the femoral head in cartilage displacing the normal bony epiphysis apparently laterally. In addition there is an upward and lateral movement of the femoral head occurring as a consequence of crushing of the dome of the bony epiphysis, with the hip subsequently becoming adducted (Fig. 7.2) In these cases there is a break in Shenton's line and arthrography shows a puddle of dye medially. An early sign of this subluxation is the appearance of a horizontal growth plate seen on the anteroposterior radiograph. This is one of the signs of the 'head-at-risk' and was originally thought to be important because of the alteration in stress forces passing through the growth plate. It has more recently been realised that the horizontal growth plate is observed when a femoral head is lying in the position of adduction and external rotation. This is an important sign present during the early and active phase of the disease and should properly be regarded as an early sign of fixed subluxation.

Measurement of subluxation has always proved difficult. This is due to the fact that the displacement of the femoral head is not lateral but anterolateral and also in cartilage. Comparatively small increases in the distance between the tear drop and the medial margin of the metaphysis (Waldenström 1934, Kemp and Boldero 1966) may be associated with considerable uncovering of the femoral head when observed arthrographically. Griffin (1980) has established a subluxation index

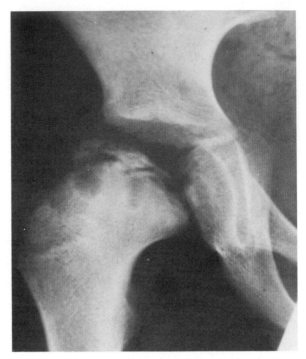

Fig. 7.8 Lateral subluxation. Child aged 6 years with Group IV disease and considerable deformity of the femoral head. There is uncovering of the femoral head laterally, with an increase in the inferomedial joint space.

helpful in prognosis but tedious in calculation. Dickens and Menelaus (1978), however, have produced a simpler measurement. This is the width of the bony epiphysis lying lateral to the margin of the bony acetabulum. This simple measurement easily reproduced and observer independent is well related to the final outcome and in the author's view the simplest of the measurements currently available.

The concept of the 'head-at-risk'

If these radiological signs of the progress of femoral head deformity are accepted, then it is possible to introduce and discuss the concept of the 'head-at-risk'. It has been noted in the study of the natural history of the groups that 90 per cent of the poor results are in Groups III and IV. In the light of the preceding discussion these poor results can be diagnosed at an early stage when they should be regarded as at-risk. These cases will be diagnosed by clinical and radiological signs.

Clinical signs

These are the older heavier child who is progressively losing movement during follow-up or who presents with an adduction contracture (Table 7.3).

Table 7.3 Signs of the head-at-risk

Clinical signs	Radiological signs
1. Heavy Child	1. Gage's sign
2. Progressive loss of movement	2. Calcification lateral to the epiphysis
3. Adduction contracture	3. Diffuse metaphyseal reaction
	4. Lateral subluxation
	5. Horizontal growth plate

Table 7.4 Results of untreated cases in relation to head at-risk factors

		Good	Fair	Poor
Group II	at-risk	12	6	2
	not at-risk	12	1	0
Group III	at-risk	5	5	3
	not at-risk	2	4	0
Group IV	at-risk	0	5	10
	not at-risk	0	0	0

Radiological signs

The five radiological signs of the head-at-risk are set out in Table 7.3. These have already been discussed in detail but may be further considered briefly.

The epiphyseal changes are Gage's sign and calcification lateral to the epiphysis. These represent early calcification and ossification occurring in the enlarged cartilagenous model and therefore are only present when femoral head deformity has already occurred, but at a stage when it is in fact reversible.

The metaphyseal changes have already been considered but represent areas of potential growth disturbance in the anterior part of the femoral head and therefore associated with femoral head deformity in the long term.

Lateral subluxation and a horizontal growth plate suggest fixed deformity and uncovering of the femoral head leading to the phenomenon of hinge abduction and therefore to progressive head deformity.

Examples of the head-at-risk are shown in Figures 7.9 and 7.10 where it will be seen that the at-risk signs occur irrespective of group. It is of interest to observe that the signs of risk are not always present in the early stages. Only after their

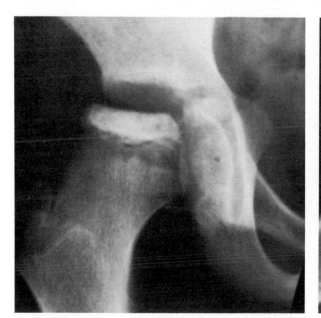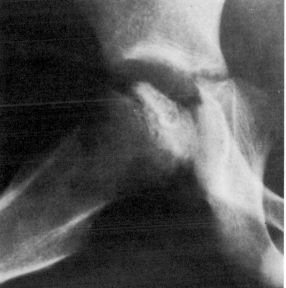

Fig. 7.9 Head-at-risk. Child aged 6 years with Group II disease. On the antero-posterior radiograph there is a horizontal growth plate, lateral subluxation and a diffuse metaphyseal change. Lateral radiograph shows 'V' sign characteristic of Group II disease.

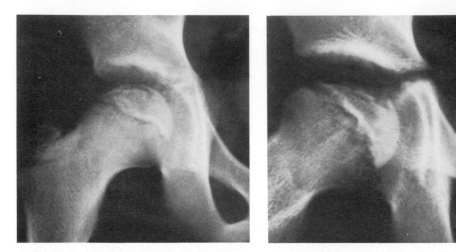

Fig. 7.10 Femoral head not-at-risk, becoming at-risk with time. (a) June 1970. Antero-posterior and lateral radiographs of Group III disease in a child of 6 years 6 months. There is no lateral subluxation, no calcification lateral to the epiphysis and no metaphyseal lesion. The growth plate is inclined to the horizontal plane.

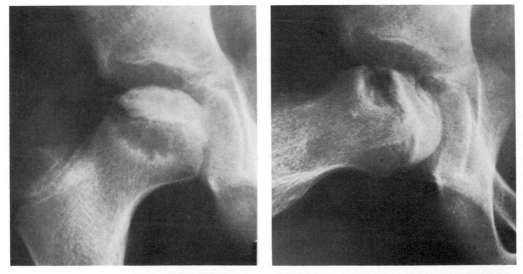

Fig. 7.10(b) October 1970. There is now a diffuse metaphyseal lesion, calcification lateral to the epiphysis, widening of the inferomedial joint space and a horizontal growth plate. These signs are now of a head-at-risk.

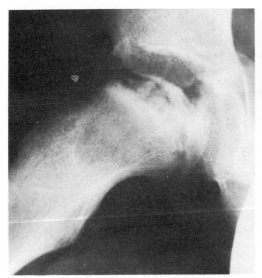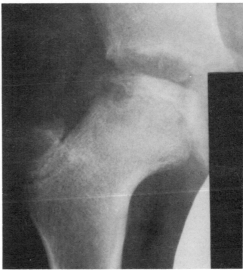

Fig. 7.10(c) August 1971. Healing is established with serious femoral head deformity present. On the lateral radiograph the change in the axis of the growth plate compared with June 1970 may be noted.

occurrence does progressive head deformity in fact occur (Fig. 7.10). This important concept allows treatment to be delayed at a stage when head at-risk signs are not present but cannot be delayed once two or more of these signs are observed.

In the untreated series, (Table 7.4), it will be seen that no case, in which a poor result ensued without treatment, did not have two or more of the at-risk signs present during the active phase of the disease. This further underlines the importance of the at-risk concept as an indication for treatment. Murphy and Marsh (1978) have reviewed the incidence of the at-risk signs confirming in their series the increasing chance of a poor result with increasing incidence of the at-risk signs. Lloyd-Roberts et al (1976) and Canario et al (1980) were the first to report a series of femoral osteotomies in which the results were compared with untreated controls. They concluded that femoral osteotomy was only of real benefit in cases where at-risk signs were present and did not alter the natural history in those cases where these factors were absent. This, therefore, provides an indication for and against operative treatment in the management of early cases.

Poor result in the long term

Although it is accepted that the signs of the head-at-risk, if present, are liable to be associated with an irregular flattened head in the short term, there are a number of femoral heads in which the initial result at the time of healing is fair but deteriorates with subsequent growth and remodelling. It has already been observed in the discussion of the long term prognosis that 11 of 75 cases followed in the long term showed a deterioration in overall result. The factors associated with this were: the age at the time of healing, the irregular head with subluxation, and the presence of a premature growth arrest in part or all of the epiphysis. If treatment is instituted at the time of healing in Groups III and IV cases bridging of the growth plate may occur (Barnes 1980). In the long term this will lead to a progressive deterioration in head shape. These findings are observed particularly when there has been an extensive metaphyseal lesion and where the femoral neck is short compared with the opposite side.

Conclusions

It is a conclusion of the evidence presented in this

Chapter that with an understanding of the morphological changes associated with progressive head deformity it is possible to define signs which are present at a stage when deformity of the femoral head is still largely cartilagenous. The presence of these clinical and radiological 'head-at-risk' signs delineate a group of patients in whom the poor results will occur without treatment. It is, however, accepted that not all cases with these signs are inevitably destined for a poor result. The converse, however, is true that in the absence of at-risk signs serious progressive femoral head deformity is unlikely to occur. Careful follow-up, however, is necessary, particularly in the older child, to ensure that at-risk signs do not appear during follow-up. It has been noted in the discussion of the long term prognosis that it is only those cases presenting an irregular flattened uncovered head at the time of healing which are destined for trouble in the short term. The clinical and radiological signs of these at-risk cases define this group. They provide therefore an absolute indiction for treatment. It must, however, be remembered that once reossification of the deformed cartilagenous model is occurring, serious alteration of pressure through this area may result in premature growth arrest actually causing a deterioration in head shape which it has been the objective of treatment to prevent.

REFERENCES

Barnes J M 1980 Premature epiphysial closure in Perthes' disease Journal of Bone and Joint Surgery 62B: 432–437

Canario A T, Williams, L, Wientroub S, Catterall A, Lloyd-Roberts G C 1980 A controlled study of the results of femoral osteotomy in severe Perthes' disease. Journal of Bone and Joint Surgery 62B: 438–440

Dickens D R V, Menelaus M B, 1978 The assessment of prognosis in Perthes' disease. Journal of Bone and Joint Surgery 60B: 189–194

Gage H C, 1933 A possible sign of Perthes' disease. British Journal of Radiology 6: 295

Griffin P P 1980 The E-L Index — value in prognosis. Paper presented at Eighth Pediatric Orthopaedic International Seminar. San Fransisco.

Kemp H S, Boldero J L 1966 Radiological changes in Perthes' disease British Journal of Radiology 39: 744–760

Lloyd-Roberts G C, Catterall A, Salamon P B, 1976 A controlled study of the indications and results of femoral osteotomy in Perthes' disease Journal of Bone and Joint Surgery 58B: 31–36

Murphy R P, Marsh H O, 1978 Incidence and natural history of head-at-risk factors in Perthes' disease. Clinical Orthopaedics and Related Research 132: 102

Waldenström H 1934 The first stage of coxa plana. Acta Orthopaedica Scandinavica 5: 1–34

8

Treatment

Introduction

It is in considering the problems of treatment of Legg-Calvé-Perthes' disease that the greatest controversies exist. There is no orthopaedic condition in which the pendulum of change has continued to swing so persistently as in the management of these children. The controversy exists because of the long duration of the disease and the fear of the late degenerative arthritis in early adult life.

Over the years the treatment protocols have varied from early mobilisation with bed rest for irritability of the joint (Calvé 1910, Perthes 1913, Schwarz 1914, Neiber 1916) to prolonged bed rest with or without the use of traction (Waldenström 1923, Danforth 1934, Mindell and Sherman 1957 and Evans 1958). The use of splints to control the position of the hip, initially of the weight-relieving type and more recently utilising the methods of containment, have had a long and persisting vogue. However, it is now generally accepted that the results of treatment utilising these splints in severe disease, especially in the child over the age of 7 years, are not satisfactory. This is particularly the case where the splints produce relief of weight without containment (Lloyd-Roberts et al 1976). More recently treatment by operative containment, using femoral or innominate osteotomy (Soeur and DeRacker 1952, Axer 1965, Salter 1973, Lloyd-Roberts et al 1976), has been reported. There is, however, persisting controversy between these methods of treatment and the mobile containment splints.

It has been an assumption of the early writers that Legg-Calvé-Perthes' disease was a uniform process in which the governing factors are those of the age and sex of the child, and the stage of the disease at which treatment was started. On this basis, when the results of treatment were assessed, matched pairs of cases were assembled based on these factors (Evans 1958, Evans and Lloyd-Roberts 1958). No attempt was made to compare these results with their untreated controls.

In a disease in which nearly 60 per cent of cases do well without treatment the conclusion reached in comparing treatment protocols which produce 62 per cent and 63 per cent good results (Evans and Lloyd-Roberts 1958) is not that both are equally effective but that neither in fact really improve the natural history of the untreated disease.

Not even the assessment of the end results of treatment can be agreed upon. These assessment protocols vary from a visual assessment Catterall 1970, Lloyd-Roberts et al 1976) to a semi-quantitative method (Eyre-Brooke 1936, Heyman and Herndon 1950, and Harrison et al 1969) to the sophisticated (Mose 1964, Curtis 1974, Klisic et al 1980). These latter methods of measurements are capable of monitoring the change in bony shape only, whereas it is known that there is a great increase in the volume of articular cartilage in this condition. The majority of assessments take little or no note of the shape of the acetabulum or of the actual congruity of the hip joint except by visual observation. It must be remembered that we are treating the hip joint of a child capable of tremendous adaptive remodelling on both sides of the joint and not just on the femoral side.

The clinician's problem, then, is to provide a treatment regime whose indications are based on an understanding of the natural history of the untreated disease and which is effective in altering its outcome. The assessment of the results must include the whole joint and not just one of its principal components.

The principles of treatment

Over the years the accepted principles of treatment have been containment of the femoral head and the relief of weight.

Containment of the femoral head within the mould of the acetabulum was a principle first reported by Eyre-Brooke (1936) although Parker, Bristow and Platt had been utilising splints in wide abduction over many years. More recently the mobile containment splints (Katz 1967, Bobechko et al 1968, Tachdjian and Jovett 1968, Harrison et al 1969, Petrie and Bitenc 1971, Roberts 1977, Purvis 1980) and containment of the femoral head by operative methods (Soeur and DeRacker 1952, Axer 1965, Lloyd-Roberts et al 1976, Salter 1973) have utilised these principles with apparently effective results.

The second principle is the relief of weight. It is logical to suggest that, when the femoral head is plastic during the active phase of the disease, reducing stress through it by the relief of weight would improve the long term outcome. Legg (1927) considering this problem wrote 'With a process suggesting weakness of bone structure it is theoretically sound to allow non weight-bearing; but in practice relief of weight-bearing in no way affects the end results'. Sundt (1949) also noted that 'Treatment directed to elimination of weight-bearing has no proved influence in the train of the morbid anatomy changes, but its application is indicated during the stage of prominent symptoms'. The reason for this failure of what at first sight appears to be effective treatment is that weight relief by bed rest or a weight-relieving caliper does not in fact seriously reduce the stresses through the joint (Trumble 1935). In addition the ring top of the weight-relieving caliper tends to encourage lateral subluxation of the femoral head (Fig. 8.1). Despite this the joint usually remains very mobile and this may account for the limited success in the Group II at-risk cases between the ages of 5 and 8 years (Catterall 1970).

When compared with untreated controls there is little to choose between the results of containment treatment in which weight-bearing is not permitted (Harrison et al 1969, Brotherton and McKib-

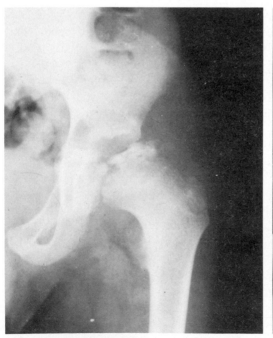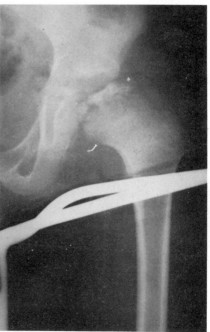

Fig. 8.1 Child aged 5 years being treated by a weight-relieving caliper. Antero-posterior radiographs taken standing with and without the weight-relieving caliper.

bin 1977) and those treatments in which it is allowed (Bobechko et al 1968, Petrie and Bitenic 1971, Salter et al 1972, Lloyd-Roberts et al 1976). In general the results are improved but particularly in the Group III cases at-risk there is no difference in the incidence of a poor result with or without the relief of weight. In Group IV, however, there is a striking difference with no poor results in the Brotherton and McKibbin series (1977). It is reasonable, therefore, to ask whether the long established principles of treatment are correct or whether there are other important principles which must be implemented to make treatment more effective, particularly in Groups III and IV cases.

The new principles

Additional principles of treatment can only be established if the process by which femoral head deformity occurs is understood. This has already been considered in some detail in the discussion of the 'poor result'. It has been concluded that femoral head deformity occurs as a result of a growth disturbance in the thickened articular cartilage and repair fibrocartilage formed as a result of the removal of crushed avascular trabecluae. This is exacerbated by initial stiffness of the hip. This growth disturbance, which is also associated with differential rates of growth of the femoral neck, leads to enlargement of the femoral head in an antero-lateral direction resulting in fixed subluxation leading to the phenomenon of hinge abduction and progressive head deformity (Fig. 3.11.f).

It may be concluded that the overriding objective of treatment must be to control the growth disturbance which occurs after epiphyseal infarction and to re-establish the normal process of ossification in the articular cartilage and fibrocartilage of the femoral head. This may be achieved with two main principles; the restoration of movement and the prevention of further ischaemia (Table 8.1).

It is known from many studies on the growing hip that for normal growth and head shape the joint must retain the normal range of movement. In the early stage of Legg-Calvé-Perthes' disease the stiffness induced by synovitis and hip irritability leads to adductor spasm and early subluxation. This can be reversed by containment of the femoral head within the mould of the acetabulum followed by mobilisation in the contained position (Table 8.1). This will allow moulding of the enlarged cartilagenous portion of the femoral head. Later in the disease there is often endochondral ossification occurring in the enlarged mass of articular cartilage (Fig. 3.11f). This new bone produces a loss of plasticity in this portion of the femoral head and improvement in the overall shape can only result from persisting growth and remodelling. In these circumstances the congruous position of the femoral head in the acetabulum may be in adduction and therefore abduction osteotomy will encourage the position of congruous incongruity and permit this long term remodelling of the femoral head to occur.

Recurrent ischaemia will result in persisting overgrowth of the articular cartilage and must be prevented if control of the growth disturbance is to be achieved. This ischaemia may be the result of recurrent synovitis producing pressure on the retinacular vessels on the side of the femoral neck or due to recurrent compression forces crushing the avascular trabecular bone intermittently interfering with its revascularisation. Forces passing through the femoral head can be substantially reduced by altering the angle of the femoral neck,

Table 8.1 The new principles of treatment

Objectives		Principles	Methods
Control of the growth disturbance by:	1. Re-establishment of normal growth	Restoration of movement	1. Containment of the femoral head
	2. Remodelling and re-ossification of thickened articular cartilage		2. Mobilisation of hip in contained position
	3. Remodelling and re-ossification of fibro-cartilage	Prevention of ischaemia	1. Prevention of synovitis
			2. Relief of stress by abduction of the hip
			3. Prevention of injury

either by abducting the leg or by varus osteotomy (Heikkinen and Puranen 1980). The optimum reduction in force is achieved with the femoral neck at 100 to 110 degrees with reference to the long axis of the body (Petrie and Bitenic 1971, Heikkinen and Puranen 1980).

If these principles are accepted it follows that treatment must be considered in three separate phases (Table 8.2). The first phase will be 'assessment and arthrography' in which the shape of the femoral head must be determined and the extent of any soft tissue contracture assessed. The second phase will be 'containment of the femoral head and mobilisation of the hip joint'. Finally there is a third phase 'maintenance of the containment until healing is established'. This will be followed by a period of growth and remodelling which should if possible persist throughout the remainder of growth. Although individual clinicians will differ slightly in the methods by which they achieve these phases, there is little difference of opinion over the practice of the first two phases of this treatment protocol. The main controversy is the maintenance of reduction until healing is established.

Table 8.2 The phases of treatment

1. Assessment and arthrography
2. Containment of the femoral head and mobilisation of the hip joint
3. Maintenance of containment until healing is established

Assessment of end results

Just as it is important to compare the results of any form of treatment with untreated controls so it is also a requirement of any form of assessment that it should reflect the long term prognosis as well as the short term. It has already been seen that following healing of the disease the remodelling process results in a 33 per cent chance of improvement in the succeeding 10 years (Table 6.2). Because of the unpredictable nature of this improvement the methods of assessment will always be relatively inaccurate. An overriding factor in the long term is that of congruency of the joint itself, particularly where there is deformity of the femoral head present. The state of congruous in-

Table 8.3 Assessment factors

1. Stage of the disease at diagnosis
2. Age and sex
3. Group
4. Signs of the head-at-risk

congruity (Curtis 1978) would seem to carry a better long term outlook than the double diameter head in which hinge abduction is occurring (Fig. 6.2c).

The very strict criteria which have been laid down by Curtis, Klisic and others and subsequently adopted by the Pediatric Orthopaedic Society deal with the sphericity of the head at the time of healing. Assessment of congruency by this method is on a visual basis. Recent papers by Perpich et al (1980) and Hall (1980) have shown that these methods and the visual assessment of Catterall (1971), Lloyd-Roberts et al (1976) do not usefully reflect the long term prognosis. Hall has shown that the measurement of head height (E.A.), a sign initially described by Catterall (1971), is a measurement which most accurately reflects the long term prognosis.

It would seem therefore, that until a better formula can be found, a visual assessment combined with a measurement of the vertical height between the growth plate and acetabulum most accurately reflects the long term outlook for these cases.

The indications for treatment

It has been seen in the discussion of the principles of treatment that therapy will be required in those cases in which the growth disturbance must be controlled because of its excessive nature. As in the management of any orthopaedic condition, the surgeon will be biased for and against a particular line of treatment as a result of the assessment of a number of factors. In Legg-Calvé-Perthes' disease these are the age and sex of the patient, the stage of the disease at diagnosis, the Group and the signs of the head-at-risk (Table 8.3).

1. The stage of the disease at diagnosis

This factor, first emphasised by Waldenström (1938), is important for three reasons. Firstly, in

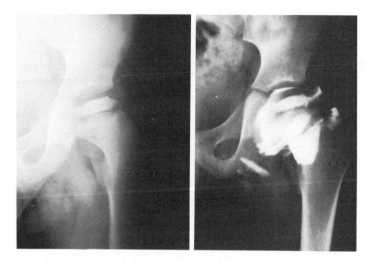

Fig. 8.2 Child aged 4 years 6 months in the active phase of the disease. There is minor uncovering of the lateral part of the epiphysis outside the line of the acetabulum. The arthrogram shows not only considerable head deformity but also the fact that the cartilagenous portion of the femoral head lies well outside the margin of the bony acetabulum.

the early stages of the disease the femoral head is usually round and for this reason offers the best opportunity for treatment if it is required. Secondly, once reabsorption of the epiphysis has commenced, with collapse of the bony structure, there may or may not be a change in the overall shape of the femoral head and this can only be established by arthrography (Fig. 8.2). Thirdly, once healing is established no further deterioration will occur in the overall shape of the femoral head (Ferguson and Howarth 1934, Westin and Thompson 1977). Treatment at this stage will not prevent further deformity, but is designed rather to improve the long term potential for remodelling by improving the congruous relationship of the femoral head to acetabulum. Femoral osteotomy undertaken at this stage may result in premature closure of part or all of the growth plate which will of course prejudice the long term result (Snyder 1975, Barnes 1980, Mindell and Sherman 1951).

2. Age and sex

These factors have already been discussed and it

has been concluded that the younger boy has a better prognosis than the older girl. The age of 6 years is considered by many authors to be the point at which the prognosis seems to change.

3. Group

The radiological signs leading to the diagnosis of Group have already been discussed in detail. The clinician is attempting by good quality radiographs, taken if necessary after a period of bed rest or traction, to assess the degree of radiological involvement of the epiphysis using the factors set out on page 47. It is accepted in the early stages, that unless a subchondral fracture line is present, it is not possible to group these patients radiologically. However, as at-risk signs are absent at this time no treatment will be required unless there are other overriding factors.

4. The signs of the head-at-risk

The five at-risk factors have already been discussed in detail. The presence of two or more of these

Table 8.4 Indications for conservative treatment

1. Group I cases
2. Groups II and III under 5 years not-at-risk
3. Groups II and III over 5 years not-at-risk
4. Cases in which severe flattening has already occurred and been demonstrated by arthrography
5. Cases in which healing is established
6. Cases demonstrating hinge abduction which cannot be corrected.

Table 8.5 Indications for definitive treatment

1. All at-risk cases
2. Group II and III cases over 7 years not-at-risk
3. Group IV cases in which severe flattening has not occurred as demonstrated by arthrography

factors in any combination adversely affects the prognosis.

With these factors in mind the indications and contraindications for treatment are set out in Tables 8.4 and 8.5. Treatment is required to control an excessive growth disturbance and will be contraindicated in those cases in which the growth disturbance is mild or in which an excessive disturbance has already occurred and cannot be altered by treatment. It will be noted that the Groups II/III spectrum of disease is subdivided by age. This is because in a younger child under 5 years it is very rare for at-risk signs to occur in the follow-up of these cases. Over the age of 7 years at-risk signs almost invariably arise during follow-up and therefore treatment should be started soon after the diagnosis has been made and before deformity has occurred. In the interval between the ages of 5 and 7 years the at-risk signs may or may not occur. Careful follow-up in this age group will be required if treatment is not undertaken when the child is first seen. It is appreciated that many of the indications for or against treatment can only be identified by arthrography which is regarded as an essential part of the assessment of these children. The assessment phase of treatment therefore has three overall aims; firstly, the extent of the growth disturbance defined by the group and at-risk signs; secondly, the establishment of the present shape of the femoral head and possible improvement in congruity by position; and thirdly the potential for remaining growth as defined by the age and sex of the patient, the patient's height in relationship to chronological and skeletal age.

The potential for remaining growth

When any treatment protocol is undertaken the subsequent result is proportional to its efficiency in preventing further femoral head deformity together with the child's ability to respond to any deformity present by a remodelling process. This remodelling process is a function of the normal growing processes present within the hip joint.

In the course of the study undertaken in 1970 the various indices described by Heyman and Herndon (1950) were monitored together with the Mose radius and the C.E. angle. Recently a study of these indices in the uninvolved hip of unilateral cases has been undertaken by Wientroub (1980) (Figs. 8.3 to 8.7). From this study, which is at the present time still incomplete, a number of observations may be drawn. There is a steady increase in the size of the femoral head with growth (Figs. 8.3 and 8.4). This occurs at approximately the same overall rate in boys and girls but is associated with a slight reduction in the ratio of epiphyseal height to width (Fig. 8.4). This suggests that an initial globular type of epiphysis becomes steadily more oval with time and hence when epiphyseal height is lost as the result of Legg-Calvé-Perthes' disease it will be more difficult for it to be regained during the course of remodelling. There is an overall increase in acetabular size with time (Fig. 8.5). In boys, however, there is steady increase in the depth of the acetabulum up to the age of 6 years, after which the ratio of acetabular height to width remains unchanged until the age of 12 years (Fig. 8.5). In girls the initial increase in depth does not occur and from the age of 4 years there is a relatively constant relationship between acetabular height and width. Similar changes are also found in the relationship between femoral neck length and width (Fig. 8.6). This very obvious difference between the sexes may go a long way to explain why the younger boy, particularly under the age of 6 years, appears to have a better prognosis than a girl of equivalent age. Fabry et al (1974) studied femoral antiversion in a number of disease processes including Legg-Calvé-Perthes' disease. They

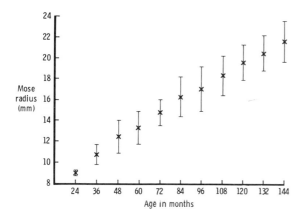

Fig. 8.3 Graph of Mose radius against time in uninvolved hips.

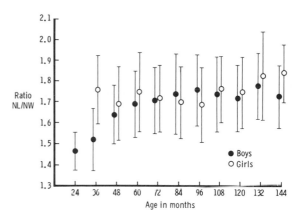

Fig. 8.6 Graph of neck ratio against time in uninvolved hips.

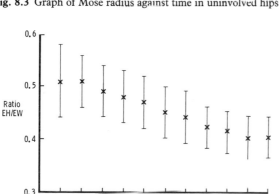

Fig. 8.4 Graph of epiphyscal ratio against time in uninvolved hips.

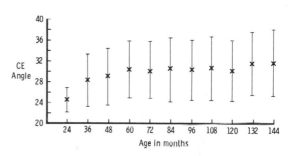

Fig. 8.7 Graph of C.E. angle against time in uninvolved hips.

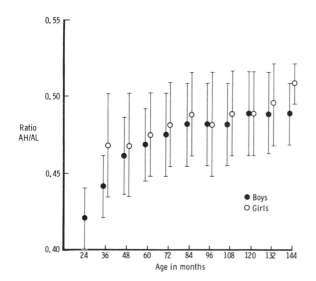

Fig. 8.5 Graph of acetabular ratio against time in uninvolved hips.

showed that on the uninvolved side of unilateral cases the angle of femoral antiversion steadily fell until the age of 8 years, after which it again increased. In normal controls this reduction of the angle of antiverson continued to occur until the adult value was achieved. Similar but more marked changes occurred on the involved side. This implies that over the age of 8 years there is a further growth disturbance in the femoral neck leading to a relative increase in the angle of antiversion and therefore an uncovering of the femoral head outside the acetabulum. This would be exacerbated by any form of metaphyseal lesion situated in the anterior and lateral part of the femoral head. Clothier (1979) has shown that the normal angle of the femoral neck is restored by growth and remodelling within 2 years after varus-rotation osteotomy in children under the age of 8 years at

the time of operation. This response is less pre-
dictable over this age.

The measurement of the C.E. angle of Wiberg
(1939) also shows unexpected results (Fig. 8.7).
The normal steady increase in this angle with time
fails to occur, suggesting that the femoral head is
not as well covered in these children as in the normal child. Minor degrees of subluxation have a
greater impact on these hips, particularly in the
older child. One of the effects of abduction might
be to improve the C.E. angle and therefore the
stability of the hip joint.

These thoughts suggest that in the younger
child there is a considerable potential for change,
particularly in the acetabulum, up to the age of 6
years to compensate for enlargement of the femoral head. However, over this age, and from the age
of 4 years in girls, these potentials for change are
not available as the result of growth, and therefore
may be required to be obtained by the treatment
protocol prescribed.

Clinical assessment

The clinical assessment of children with Legg-
Calvé-Perthes' disease begins with a careful history and examination. Particular attention is paid
to the duration of symptoms and their onset.
There may or may not have been a history of
trauma in the ensuing weeks before symptoms
occur or an episode of an acute hip irritability.
The limp is typically intermittent and this is
another factor which may help to date the onset of
symptoms. The child's general health should be
investigated, particularly any previous illnesses or
operations for hernia or genito-urinary disease. It
is unusual to obtain a family history of this condition and its presence would suggest a Perthes-like
change. The illnesses and operations in the parents and other first degree relatives should be
noted.

After a full general examination height and
weight are noted. The child is then observed walking and the nature of the associated limp assessed.
The hips are next examined, comparing the range
of movement present in the involved with the
opposite hip and establishing the presence and nature of any joint contracture. Leg lengths are mea-
sured. The knees and feet should also be ex-

amined as it will be remembered that approximately 20 per cent of the children may have
Köhler's disease of the navicular. The clinical sign
of this condition is stiffness of subtaloid movement.

Plain radiographs are now taken in the antero-
posterior and Lauenstein lateral views of the joint.
If the diagnosis has already been established and
there is any serious restriction of hip movement
the child should be rested and these radiographs
only obtained when the hip has loosened up.
Radiographs of the hands to establish the bone age
of the child and lateral radiographs of the feet are
also taken. All these radiographs must be carefully
studied to establish the radiological grouping, the
stage of the disease, and the presence of head-at-
risk signs.

With the knowledge of the age and sex of the
patient, their height and weight, the presence of
stiffness or joint contracture and the radiological
signs just discussed, the clinician is now able to
advise on treatment using the indications that have
been previously defined. In those cases in which
there is a good range of movement, and radiological features suggest a good prognosis, no treatment
apart from out-patient supervision is advised and
the child is re-assessed clinically and radiologically
every three months. In those cases in which serious treatment is being considered further assessment will be required in the form of an examination under anaesthetic with arthrography.

Examination under anaesthetic and arthrography

This examination is conveniently conducted in the
Department of Radiology but may equally well be
undertaken in any part of the hospital where an
image intensifier is available. It is important to
stress that this is a careful examination of the child
who is anaesthetised and is best thought of as
'Thinking with a needle'. The range of movement
under anaesthetic is carefully assessed and compared with the pre-operative state to separate joint
contracture from postural deformity and spasm.
Forty-five per cent hypaque is now injected into
the hip joint using image intensification in order to
establish the shape of the cartilagenous part of the
femoral head and its congruency with the acetabulum. Movements of the hip are now observed on

the image intensifier and changes in the congruity between the femoral head and acetabulum noted as the hip is moved in the abduction and adduction range and also in flexion and extension. (Fig. 8.8). It is commonly noted that the most congruent position between the femoral head and acetabulum is in the position of adduction (Fig. 8.8d) and this confirms the observation that for much of the time the hip tends to lie in the adducted position. Provided there is no femoral head deformity it will be seen that as the leg is abducted the femoral head rotates into the acetabulum so that the majority of the head is covered in the position of abduction and internal rotation. This movement is a combination of rotation and hinging. On other occasions, however, the femoral head is best contained if flexion is added to the position of abduction and internal rotation. These two positions provide the indications for femoral and innominate osteotomy (Table 8.6). Having noted these observations on the image intensifier, routine films in neutral, adduction, abduction and internal rotation, and flexion abduction and internal rotation, together with laterals in the neutral and best contained position, are taken for further study and for record purposes (Fig. 8.8).

Sometimes on abduction no containment of the femoral head is possible and it is noted that on attempting abduction the femoral head hinges on the lateral lip of the acetabulum (Fig. 8.9). This phenomenon, called "Hinge Abduction", has already been discussed and is a contraindication to containment by abduction and internal rotation unless the process of hinging can be reversed and the whole femoral head contained within the mould of the acetabulum. In these cases congruity is present with the leg in the adducted position. Particularly, when healing is established, this is an indication for abduction osteotomy (Table 8.6).

In the late case where healing is either established or already complete an arthrogram will be helpful in elucidating the cause of pain. The radiographs may demonstrate the presence of an osteocartilagenous loose body or an abnormality of the limbus which may in fact be torn and present with the clinical syndrome of instability.

At the conclusion of this examination the shape of the femoral head and any changes in its congruity with the acetabulum during the course of

Table 8.6 Results of arthrography

Arthrographic finding	Operation
1. Containment obtained in:	
a. Abduction and internal rotation	Femoral osteotomy (varus and rotation)
b. Flexion and abduction and internal rotation	Innominate osteotomy
2. Containment not improved	No treatment
3. Hinge abduction	Abduction osteotomy

movement will be established. During the active phases of the disease containment treatment by whatever method is chosen will be indicated in those cases in which the cartilagenous portion of the femoral head becomes fully contained within the mould of the acetabulum. The position of congruity will determine the form of treatment advocated (Table 8.6). Severe femoral head deformity associated with Hinge Abduction would be regarded as a contraindication to containment treatment. In these cases abduction osteotomy would improve the chances of satisfactory long term remodelling.

The technique of arthrography. It is important in obtaining good quality arthrograms that as little as possible of the dye injected is extraversated outside the joint. It is particularly important if the anterior and lateral aspect of the joint is to be examined that there should be no extraversated dye in this area. It is therefore preferable to inject the hip via a needle approaching the joint from the perineal aspect (Fig. 8.10). This is undertaken with the hip in the flexed and abducted position, and the needle is inserted just posterior to the tendon of adductor longus and just medial to the line of the anterior superior iliac spine. The needle should make contact with bone at the junction of the posterior and medial aspect of the metaphysis. Sufficient dye (45 per cent hypaque) should be injected to outline the joint surfaces (3–4 cc). The injection of too much dye will result in failure to visualise anything but the surface of the joint and valuable information, particularly on the thickness of the articular cartilage, will be lost.

If there is considerable deformity of the femoral head it may be better to approach the joint from an anterior aspect. The needle is aimed to reach

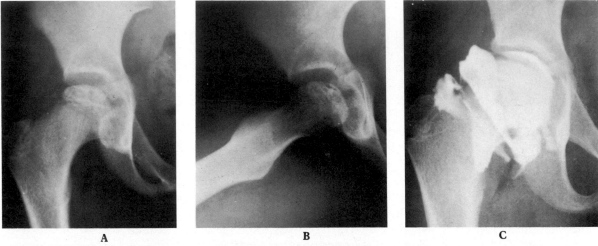

A   B   C

Fig. 8.8 Child aged 6 years 6 months with Group III Perthes' disease. (**a** and **b**) Antero-posterior and lateral radiographs confirming the Group III appearance. A subchondral fracture line reaches into the posterior part of the head. (**c**) The arthrogram showing minor incongruity with the leg in the neutral position.

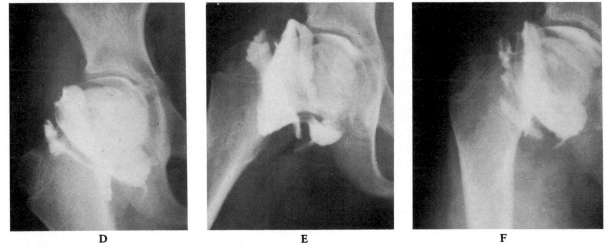

D   E   F

Fig. 8.8(d) Congruity with the leg in 20 degrees of adduction. (**e**) The position in abduction and internal rotation showing containment of the femoral head and particularly the enlarged lateral cartilagenous part. (**f**) The position in flexion abduction and internal rotation showing that the containment is not as good as in abduction and internal rotation.

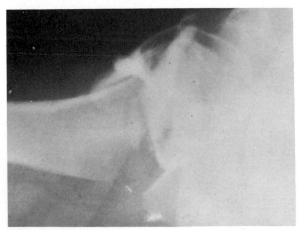

Fig. 8.8(g) The Smith Petersen lateral view showing the anterior uncovering of the femoral head and the deformity of its anterior half.

G

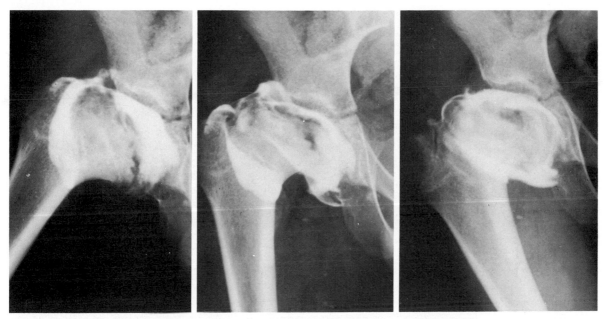

Fig. 8.9 Arthrogram of a child with severe femoral head deformity. In the centre radiograph the leg is in the neutral position and the lateral acetabular margin in indenting the lateral part of the femoral head. The radiograph on the left shows the phenomenon of hinge abduction. On the right, congruity of this hip joint is obtained with the leg in 20 degrees of abduction; the dent in the lateral margin of the femoral head may be observed.

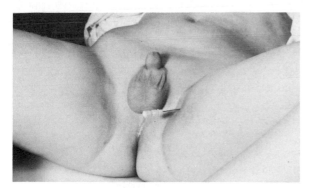

Fig. 8.10 Position for arthrography by perineal route.

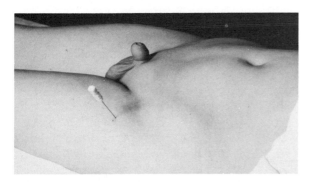

Fig. 8.11 Position for arthrography by the anterior routes.

the junction of the lateral aspect of the epiphysis with the femoral neck (Fig. 8.11).

Containment of the femoral head and mobilisation of the hip joint

Once it has been decided to proceed with containment treatment during the active phase of the disease the second phase of treatment is now undertaken; the containment of the femoral head and mobilisation. Cylinder plasters are applied to both legs with the knees in approximately 30 degrees of flexion. An adjustable bar (Fig. 8.12) is applied to these plasters with the uninvolved leg in approximately the neutral position of rotation and 20 degrees of abduction and the involved hip in as much abduction and internal rotation as the patient, while awake, will comfortably tolerate. Thereafter and on a daily basis the screws are loosened and the involved leg abducted and internally rotated until the fully contained position of the femoral head has been achieved. This position will have been defined at the time of arthrography. If during the course of this treatment the hip becomes irritable no further change in position is made until movement has returned. This will

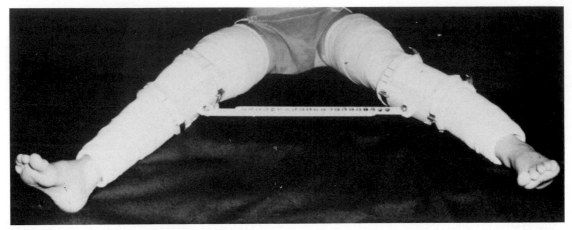

Fig. 8.12 The adjustable Broomstick plaster.

usually occur in 24 to 48 hours. On this regime it is found that the femoral head is contained within the acetabulum and the hip mobile in the flexion extension range in approximately 2 weeks. This position is then checked radiologically to be sure that it corresponds with the arthrographic appearances. If there is any doubt about the position of containment the arthrogram is repeated.

It is possible using this technique to reverse mild degrees of hinge abduction (Fig. 8.13).

The maintenance of containment until healing is established

It is in this aspect and phase of treatment that the greatest controversies over management exist. The main arguments centre on whether the contained position should be maintained by splintage or operative means and whether this should be combined with weight relief.

At first sight the gulf between the operative and orthotic methods of management would seem to be unbridgable. However, the majority of advocates for treatment by splintage reserve this method for the younger child with the milder form of the disease. They reserve operative treatment either for a failure of this primary management or for the older child with more serious disease. The age of 7 years is regarded by some as the upper limit for treatment by splintage. It is relevant to observe that in boys this is approximately the age at which the potential for change in growth in the femoral neck and acetabulum is altering.

The ideals of effective treatment would be to shorten the duration of the disease process by biologically triggering the healing mechanism; reduce lateral uncovering of the femoral head by containing it within the mould of the acetabulum and encouraging movement; permit full activity and weight-bearing; cause no injury to the growth plate; and finally be ethically acceptable (Table 8.7). Neither treatment by operation or splintage can achieve all these objectives and it is pertinent therefore to compare and contrast the potentials of these treatments and the common points between them.

Table 8.7 Aims of effective treatment

1. Shorten the duration of disease
2. Biologically trigger the healing process
3. Reduce lateral uncovering
4. Restore movement
5. Permit full activity and weight-bearing
6. Cause no injury to the growth plate
7. Be ethically acceptable

Orthotic treatment has the immediate advantage of almost no period of time in hospital and, particularly, no operation. The methods of treatment are by and large cumbersome and although some children do not require the use of crutches the majority are sufficiently incapacitated by their splint for the use of crutches to be mandatory for reasonable activity. Extravagent claims are, however, made for the mobility of these children. One of the immediate difficulties in management concerns the time at which the splint is removed With operative treatment the splint or hip spica is

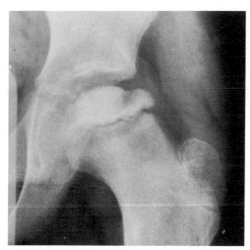

Fig. 8.13(a) April 1972. A child aged 10 years 6 months with established Group III disease. The femoral head is uncovered outside the line of the acetabulum. There is a horizontal growth plate and a diffuse metphayseal reaction.

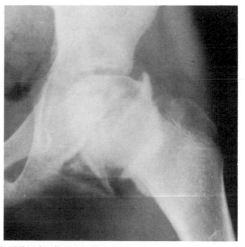

Fig. 8.13(b) April 1972. The arthrogram showing the dent on the lateral aspect of the femoral head, the whole of which is contained within the mould of the acetabulum in abduction and internal rotation.

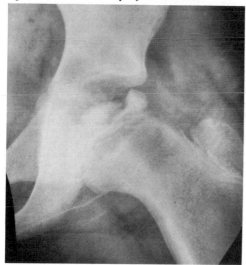

Fig. 8.13(c) May 1972. Following mobilisation in an adjustable Broomstick plaster, the child has a full range of flexion and extension with the femoral head well seated within the acetabulum.

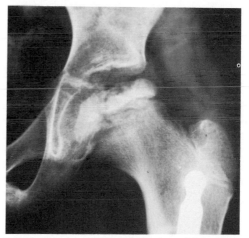

Fig. 8.13(d) November 1972. Healing is established following femoral osteotomy.

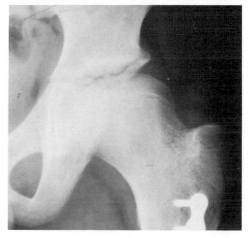

Fig. 8.13(e) October 1976. Healing is complete. The dent previously noted on arthrography has remodelled.

discarded when the osteotomy is united. A similar end point is not defined so easily with conservative treatment in which splints are utilised. If it is accepted that treatment may be discontinued as soon as healing is established (Ferguson and Howarth 1934), then in the short term it has been shown that there will be no deleterious effect. Evidence is not available, however, on whether there are long term consequences for growth and remodelling as the result of altering the stress through the hip at this stage. There is no evidence to suggest that such splintage shortens the duration of disease. In the majority of the splints in current use the knee is immobilised in order to control the position of the hip and this will inevitably lead in some cases to stiffness which may or may not have a long lasting disadvantage. Particularly in those splints where weight relief is also required (Harrison et al, 1969), the length of the legs must be carefully watched and regular hip exercises encouraged if serious shortening is to be avoided. The splint will also require regular checking in order to establish that containment of the femoral head is being maintained.

Operative treatment also has advantages and disadvantages. Provided the child is carefully assessed and the position of containment established then realignment osteotomy, either above or below the hip, can maintain this containment. This position is maintained throughout the healing and remodelling phases of the disease. The varus, particularly, will relieve stress through the femoral head permitting, therefore, remodelling to continue through the period of growth (Somerville 1971). By comparison with untreated controls femoral osteotomy will shorten the duration of the disease, particularly to the onset of healing (Table 8.8). This observation is important as with the onset of healing no further deterioration will occur in the shape of the femoral head, and the

remodelling phase can commence. Osteotomy does, however, have two serious disadvantages. By the nature of the realignment process femoral osteotomy will produce shortening. In the majority of cases this is between half and three quarters of an inch following operation. Although this is obviously a problem in the short term, experience has shown that it will correct itself as the result of growth and remodelling in the proximal femur in the course of the next two years. Canario et al (1980) and Clothier (1979) have shown that after two years the majority of children have a quarter of an inch or less of true shortening. The exception to this rule is in children over the age of 8 years. Here this spontaneous correction of the shortening is less reliable and if the varus produced as a result of osteotomy is excessive a progressive coxa vara may occasionally ensue. Persisting varus will also produce a relative overgrowth of the greater trochanter. The second disadvantage of operation is an injury to the growth plate. This problem has already been discussed in the analysis of the poor result. The conclusion has been made that it is liable to occur when surgery is undertaken in the child with Groups III and IV disease, particularly in the healing phase.

It may be concluded therefore that during this phase of treatment there are advantages and disadvantages of both forms of therapy in the younger child with at-risk signs. In the older child, with at-risk signs, however, the place of containment treatment by splintage would seem less well established and many clinicians would advise operation. The major residual problem which still confronts the clinician is the problem of weight relief. In the past it has been a principle of treatment that weight should not be permitted through the hip during the active phase of the disease. However, the experience of containment splints in which weight-bearing is permitted would suggest that this is not always the case. Brotherton and McKibbin (1977) reporting the long term results of the A.O. Parker series have shown that although the results in the Group III cases at-risk treated by bed rest with Broomstick plasters are not seriously different from those treated by femoral osteotomy, in the Group IV cases there are no poor results. This is in contrast

Table 8.8 Duration of disease (months)

		Healing	Healed
II —	Untreated	9.4	27.8
	Osteotomy	8.0	25.8
III —	Untreated	14.6	32.5
	Osteotomy	11.6	32.0
IV —	Untreated	17.4	41.6
	Osteotomy	14.8	35.8

with all other forms of therapy currently reported. The Group IV cases treated by femoral osteotomy (Lloyd-Roberts et al 1976) show 35 per cent poor results. In this series containment femoral osteotomy was not preceded by a phase of mobilisation prior to operation. In the prospective series to be discussed in the next chapter this factor has been added to the treatment protocol with a corresponding improvement in the incidence of poor results in the Group IV cases. It would seem, therefore, that the principle of restoration of movement to the hip joint may be more important than the relief of weight. Both these principles have been applied in the management of the Brotherton and McKibbin series although the factor of weight relief has been regarded as being more important.

The technique of femoral osteotomy

This operation is performed under general anaesthetic. A unit of blood compatible with the patient should be available for transfusion in the case of excessive blood loss.

The operation is undertaken with the patient in the supine position (Fig. 8.14). An oblique incision is made from the posterior aspect of the tip of the trochanter laterally down the thigh. The subcutaneous tissues and fascia lata are incised in the line of their fibres. The trochanteric bursa is opened on the antero-lateral aspect of the femur and the fatty tissue lying anteriorly dissected from

the inter-trochanteric line. A 'T' shaped incision is made in the attachment of the vastus medialis with its longitudinal part of the 'T' in the posterior third of this attachment (Fig. 8.15). A subperiosteal exposure is made to the upper part of the femur and four spikes inserted, the most proximal and medial of which is placed to demonstrate the base of the femoral neck.

The leg is placed so that the femoral head is in the contained position of abduction and internal rotation. A guide wire is inserted into the lateral aspect of the upper shaft and passed up the femoral neck and parallel to the ground. A drill hole is made in the anterior shaft just above the proposed site of femoral osteotomy and will act as the second screw in a four hole plate (Fig. 8.16). The bone is divided exactly at right angles to the shaft (Fig. 8.17).

The subperiosteal exposure of the lower fragment is completed and the bone rotated so that the patella is in the neutral position and the leg parallel to the opposite side. When abduction and internal rotation have been corrected, the distal shaft is displaced a little medial on the proximal fragment to allow for better biomechanical remodelling. This has the effect of apparently reducing the size of the opening wedge that is required for correction. The osteotomy is stabil-

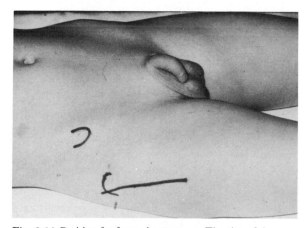

Fig. 8.14 Position for femoral osteotomy. The tips of the anterior superior iliac spine and greater trochanter are marked and the line of the skin incision indicated.

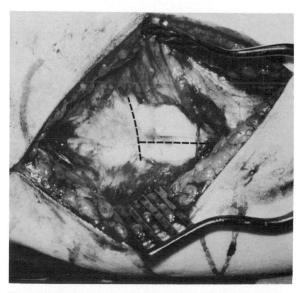

Fig. 8.15 The exposure of vastus lateralis and glutius medius. The 'T' shaped incision is indicated.

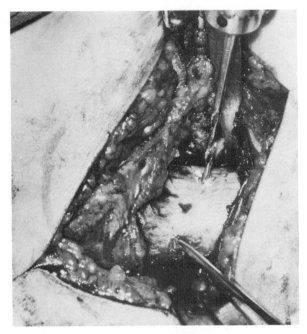

Fig. 8.16 Drilling the first screw hole after the insertion of the guide wire.

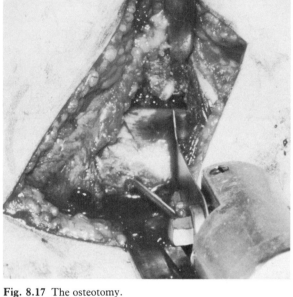

Fig. 8.17 The osteotomy.

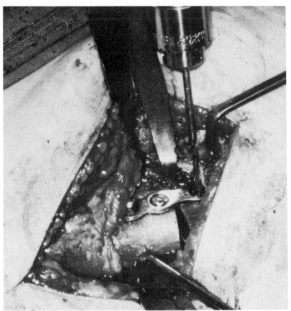

Fig. 8.18 Drilling the first hole on the distal fragment. The drill is at right angles to the floor.

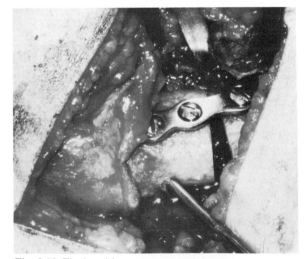

Fig. 8.19 Final position.

ised using a four hole plate. The first screw is passed through the second screw hole in the four hole plate and inserted into the drill hole previously made. Care is taken to maintain the rotational correction required by holding the patella in the neutral position while the plate is secured to the distal fragment (Fig. 8.18). At this stage minor corrections of varus and valgus angulation are still possible but the rotation is fixed. The proximal screw is inserted (Fig. 8.19). The wound is closed in layers.

Post-operatively a plaster hip spica is applied

and is retained for a total period of 9 weeks. At this stage the plaster is removed and the child mobilised. It is not uncommon for crutches to be required for the first two to three weeks but thereafter they may be rapidly discarded as mobility is regained.

The assessment of the late case

Unfortunately many children present in the later phases of the disease with advanced femoral head deformity. Some of these children have pain but the majority have a persisting limp. This is due to shortening, resulting from stiffness and fixed adduction of the hip. Most clinicians now agree that treatment by splintage will not improve the end result in this situation. A number of operative procedures, including chielectomy or the Garceau procedure, the Chiari operation, trochanteric epiphysiodesis and abduction osteotomy have been advised. The clinician, therefore, will require to have indications and contraindications to all these procedures.

If these children are left untreated at this stage the majority will continue to limp although the limp will become less obvious with time. It is unusual for them to have serious pain during adolescence. Grossbard (1981) in a review of the causes of pain in this adolescent group has established four aetiologies; an osteochondritic loose body, hinge abduction, an injury to the acetabular labrum and discomfort due to overgrowth of the greater trochanter. Simple uncovering of the femoral head was not in itself found to be a cause of pain.

It is in the light of this natural history that the various operative procedures must be considered. It has been established that for good long term remodelling a congruous relationship is required between the femoral head and the acetabulum with the leg in the neutral weight-bearing position. It is also known that when severe deformity of the femoral head is present there is considerable enlargement of both femoral head and acetabulum. The theory has been advanced by Pauwels (1951) that early degenerative changes are the consequence of high pressure loading of a local area of the femoral head. If there is a relative increase in total hip joint surface then there is a correspond-

ing reduction in force per unit area provided that the greater part of the joint can be made weight-bearing in the neutral position. In these circumstances chielectomy or the Garceau procedure which excises approximately a third of the lateral aspect of the femoral head has the advantage of removing the cause of hinge abduction but the disadvantage of seriously reducing the load-bearing area of the joint. The long term results of this procedure are not available and it will be interesting to observe the incidence of osteoarthritis compared with the known long term results of untreated cases. The Chiari operation will not seriously alter the process of hinge abduction but will reduce the abductor level arm and improve the cover of the lateral aspect of the femoral head. The short term results of this procedure are encouraging but the long term consequences must be awaited. This operation or a lateral shelf acetabuloplasty (Van der Heyden and Van Tongerloo 1980) would seem indicated during the healing phases of the disease in the older child when considerable femoral head deformity has occurred and where abduction osteotomy is considered unsuitable. If, however, the cause of the pain is a tear of the acetabular labrum, the Chiari procedure by operating in this area may remove this source of pain.

If it is accepted that the major source of pain in these late cases is the consequence of hinge abduction then it is logical to correct this, as in the adult (Bombelli 1976), by abduction osteotomy. At the time of arthrography it is possible to show that these hips are congruent in adduction and have an arc of adduction beyond this point of congruity. Femoral osteotomy designed to realign the leg in the middle of this arc of movement will allow this congruent position to be obtained when the patient is weight-bearing and stop the phenomenon of hinging, thereby allowing a better chance for remodelling. This operation which has the great advantage of simplicity does not remove bone from the femoral head and therefore does not seriously alter the forces within the joint. In the short term (Fig. 8.20) it is surprising how much the femoral head will round up with remodelling, but it is again too soon for the long term results for this procedure to be known.

The reduction of the compressive forces on the lateral lip of the acetabulum induced by the hing-

Fig. 8.20 Treatment by abduction osteotomy. Child aged 7 years with healing Group IV disease.

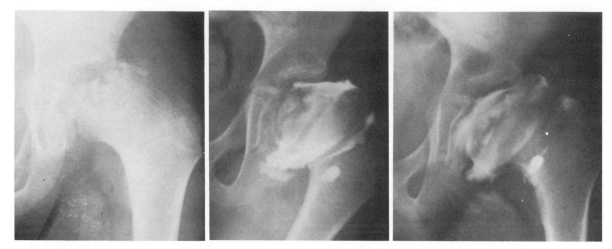

Fig. 8.20(a) September 1977. There was a flexion/adduction contracture. Antero-posterior radiograph showing gross deformity with lateral uncovering.

Fig. 8.20(b) The arthrogram showing hinge abduction with congruency in adduction.

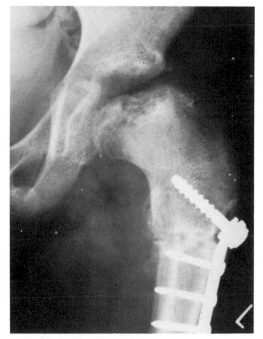

Fig. 8.20(c) January 1979. 9 months following abduction femoral osteotomy.

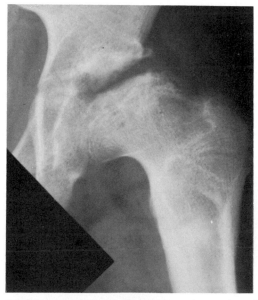

Fig. 8.20(d) September 1980. Healing is nearly complete. The femoral head is becoming better contained and the lateral lip of the acetabulum continues to develop.

ing phenomenon will allow a resumption of the normal growth processes in this part of the joint with a resumption of lateral growth, and therefore better cover of the femoral head (Fig. 8.20).

REFERENCES

Axer A 1965 Subtrochanteric osteotomy in the treatment of Perthes' disease. Journal of Bone and Joint Surgery 47B: 489–499

Barnes J M 1980 Premature epiphysial closure in Perthes' disease. Journal of Bone and Joint Surgery 62B: 432–437

Bobechko W P, McLaurin C A, Motlock W M 1968 Toronto orthosis for Legg-Perthes' disease. Artificial Limbs 12: 36

Bombelli R 1976 Osteoarthritis of the hip. Pathogenesis and consequent therapy. Springer-Verlag, Berlin, Heidelberg, New York.

Brotherton B J, McKibbin B 1977 Perthes' disease treated by prolonged recumbancy and femoral head containment, a long term appraisal. Journal of Bone and Joint Surgery 59B: 14

Calvé J 1910 Sur une forme particulare de pseudo-coxalgia greffee sur des deformations caracteristiques de l'extremite superiure due femur Revue de Chirurgie 30: 54–84

Canario A T, Williams L, Wientroub S, Catterall A, Lloyd-Roberts G C 1980 A controlled study of the results of femoral osteotomy in severe Perthes' disease. Journal of Bone and Joint Surgery 62B: 438–440

Catterall A 1970 Personal observations

Catterall A 1971 The natural history of Perthes' disease. Journal of Bone and Joint Surgery 53B: 37–53

Clothier J C 1979 The behaviour of upper femoral osteotomies performed for Perthes' disease. Journal of Bone and Joint Surgery 61B: 517

Curtis B H, Gunther S F, Gossling H R, Siegfried W P 1974 Treatment for Legg-Perthes disease with the Newington ambulation and abduction brace. Journal of Bone and Joint Surgery 56A: 1135

Curtis B H 1978 Personal communication

Danforth M S 1934 The treatment of Legg-Calve-Perthes' disease without weight bearing. Journal of Bone and Joint Surgery 16: 516–534

Evans D L 1958 Legg-Calvé-Perthes' disease. A study of late results. Journal of Bone and Joint Surgery 40B: 168–181

Evans D L, Lloyd-Roberts G C 1958 Treatment in Legg-Calvé-Perthes' disease. A comparison of inpatient and outpatient methods. Jorunal of Bone and Joint Surgery 40B: 182–189

Eyre-Brooke A L 1936 Osteochondritis deformans coxae juvenilis or Perthes' disease. The results of treatment by traction in recumbancy British Journal of Surgery 24: 166–182

Fabry G, MacEwen G D, Shands A R 1973 Torsion of the femur. Journal of Bone and Joint Surgery 55A: 1726

Ferguson A B, Howarth M B 1934 A study of coxa plana and related conditions of the hip. Journal of Bone and Joint Surgery 16: 781

Garceau G, Rapp G, Lidge R T 1973 Coxa plana (A surgical approach). Journal of Bone and Joint Surgery 55A: 1313

Grossbard G 1981 Personal communication

Hall G 1980 Some observations on Perthes' disease. Robert Jones Prize Essay of the British Orthopaedic Association.

Harrison M H M, Turner M H, Nicholson F J 1969 Coxa plana. Results of a new form of splinting. Journal of Bone and Joint Surgery 51A: 1057–1069

Heikkinen E, Puranen J 1980 Evaluation of femoral osteotomy in the treatment of Legg-Calvé-Perthes' disease. Clinical Orthopaedics and Related Research 150: 60–68

Heyman C H, Herndon C H 1950 Legg-Perthes' disease. A method for measurement of the roentgenographic results. Journal of Bone and Joint Surgery 32A: 767

Katz J F 1967 Conservative treatment of Legg-Calve-Perthes' disease. Journal of Bone and Joint Surgery 49A: 1043–1051

Klisic P, Blazevic U, Seferovic O 1980 Approach to treatment of Legg-Calve-Perthes' disease. Clinical Orthopaedics 150: 54–59

Legg A T 1927 End results of coxa plana. Journal of Bone and Joint Surgery 9: 26–36

Lloyd-Roberts G C, Catterall A, Salamon P B 1976 A controlled study of the indications and results of femoral osteotomy in Perthes' disease. Journal of Bone and Joint Surgery 58B: 31–36

Mindell E R, Sherman M S 1951 Late results in Legg-Perthes' disease. Journal of Bone and Joint Surgey 33A: 1–23

Mose K 1964 Legg-Calvé-Perthes' disease — results of treatment. A comparison between three methods of conservative treatment. Copenhagen Universitetsforlaget 1964

Neiber O 1916 Ueber osteochondritis deformans. Coxae juvenilis (Perthes) Zietschr fur Orthopaedic Chirurgie 35: 301

Pauwels F 1951 Des affections de la hanche d'origine mechanique et de leur traitement par l'osteotomie d'adduction. Rev. Chir. Orthop. 37: 22

Perpich M, Kruse D, McBeath A A 1980 Long term follow-up of Legg-Calvé-Perthes disease treated with hip spica cast. Paper presented at Meeting of American Orthopaedica Association, Honolulu, 1980

Perthes G C 1913 Osteochondritis deformans juvenilis Archives fur Klinische Chirurgie 101: 779–807

Petrie J G, Bitenc I 1971 The abduction weight bearing treatment in Legg-Perthes' disease. Journal of Bone and Joint Surgery 53B: 54

Purvis J M, Dimon J H, Meehan P C, Lovell W W 1980 Preliminary experience with Scottish Rite Hospital abduction orthosis for Legg-Perthes' disease Clinical Orthopaedics and Related Research 150: 49–53

Roberts J M 1977 Ambulatory abduction brace for Legg-Perthes' disease First International Symposium Legg-Perthes' Syndrome. Los Angeles, p 99

Salter R B, Rang M, Bell M 1972 The scientific basis for innominate osteotomy in the treatment of Legg-Perthes' disease. Annals of Royal College of Physicians and Surgery of Canada 62:

Salter R B 1973 Legg-Perthes' disease — treatment by innominate osteotomy. American Academy of Orthopaedic Surgeons. Instructional Course Lectures 22: 309–316

Schwarz E 1914 quoted by Edgren W. Acta Orthopaedica Scandinavica Supp. 84: p 25

Snyder C R 1975 Legg-Perthes' disease in the young hip — does it necessarily do well? Journal of Bone and Joint Surgery 57A: 751–758

Soeur R, DeRacker C 1952 L'aspect anatomo-pathologique de l'osteochondrite e les theories pathogeniques qui s'y rapportent. Acta Orthopaedics Belge 18: 57

Somerville E W 1971 Perthes' disease of the hip. Journal of Bone and Joint Surgery 53B: 639–649

Sundt H 1949 Further investigations respecting mature coxae-Calve-Legg-Perthes' disease with special regard to prognosis and treatment. Acta Chirugica Scandinavica Suppl. 148

Tachdjian M O, Jovett L D 1968 Trilateral socket hip abduction orthosis for treatment of Legg-Perthes' disease. Journal of Bone and Joint Surgery 50A: 1272

Trumble H C 1935 Weight bearing instruments for walking. British Medical Journal i: 1010

Van der Heyden A M, Van Tongerloo R B 1980 Shelf operation in Perthes' disease. Paper presented to Continental Meeting of Dutch, Norvic and British Orthopaedic Association, October 1980

Waldenström H 1923 On coxa plana: osteochondritis deformans coxa juvenilis. Leggs disease, Maladie de Calvé, Perthes Krankheit. Acta Chirugica Scandinavica 55: 577–590

Waldenström H 1938 The first stages of Coxa plana. Journal of Bone and Joint Surgery 20: 559–566

Westin G W, Thompson G H, 1977 Legg-Calvé-Perthes' disease. The results of discontinuing treatment in reformative phase. First International Symposium on Legg-Calve-Perthes Syndromes, Los Angeles 1977

Wiberg G 1939 Studies on dysplastic acetabula and congenital subluxation of the hip joint, with special reference to the complication of osteoarthritis. Acta Chirugica Scandinavica Suppl. 58:

Wientroub S 1980 Personal communication.

9

The results of treatment

Introduction

In the preceding chapters of this book the clinical features and morbid anatomy have been discussed together with the radiological features of this condition. On the basis of these thoughts the principles of treatment have been established and a protocol suggested. These theories and principles can only be tested by reviewing a series of cases in which they have formed the basis of treatment. Such a series would answer the question 'will treatment only help selected cases?'.

Clinical material

Between 1971 and 1977 84 cases of Legg-Calvé-Perthes' disease were referred to the Paediatric Orthopaedic Departments of the Royal National Orthopaedic Hospital and the Charing Cross Group of Hospitals. Of these 19 were bilateral and 14 were in girls. The average age at the presentation was 6.2 years with an average follow-up of 5.6 years (Tables 9.1 and 9.2). All were diagnosed as having Legg-Calvé-Perthes' disease in the active or healing phases. Of the 103 hips available for study 14 had been excluded. In 3 of these, operative treatment was advised but refused by the patient. These cases developed a poor result. In the remaining hips the child had received considerable treatment, usually in the

Table 9.1 1980 survey

84 patients: 70 boys, 14 girls	
Bilateral cases	19
Average age at presentation	6.2 years
Average follow-up	5.6 years (min. 3.0 years; max 9 years)

Table 9.2 1980 Survey

		Group				Total	
		I	II	III	IV	No.	%
Conservative	Early untreated	17	8	2	3	30	(34)
	Healing	0	6	6	7	19	(21)
Definitive	Osteotomy	0	12	21	7	40	(45)
		17	26	29	17	89	(100)

form of bed rest or a weight-relieving caliper and were referred late in the disease process for further assessment. In all cases healing was established and considerable deformity of the femoral head present. Because of this, surgical treatment was considered contraindicated and they have, therefore, been excluded. Of the remaining 89 hips (Table 9.2), 70 were in the active phase of the disease and 19 in the healing stages, but recently diagnosed. It was considered that these cases were similar to those reported in other series and represented disease for whose treatment I was primarily responsible.

Methods of treatment

After clinical assessment a decision was made as to whether the case would be treated conservatively without treatment, or definitively by operation. The indications and contra-indications to definitive treatment are set out in Tables 9.3 and 9.4 and are the same as those previously discussed. Arthrography was undertaken in all cases in whom operative treatment was being considered or where healing was established in the presence of some epiphyseal deformity to see if congruity could be improved. Forty cases were treated by

Table 9.3 Indications for conservative treatment

1. Group I cases
2. Groups II and III under 5 years not-at-risk
3. Groups II and III over 5 years not-at-risk
4. Cases in which severe flattening has already occurred and been demonstrated by arthrography
5. Cases in which healing is established
6. Cases demonstrating hinge abduction which cannot be corrected.

Table 9.4 Indications for definitive treatment.

1. All at-risk cases
2. Groups II and III cases over 7 years not at-risk
3. Group IV cases in which severe flattening has not occurred as demonstrated by arthrography.

operation, of which 27 had femoral osteotomies and 13 innominate osteotomies. Femoral osteotomy was indicated in those cases where the femoral head was best contained in abduction and internal rotation (Fig. 9.1, 9.3) and innominate osteotomy where flexion was in addition required to the abduction and internal rotation (Fig. 9.2). When operative treatment was advised, the hip was mobilised pre-operatively in the contained position using the adjustable Broomstick plaster. Following operation the hip was immobilised in a plaster spica for a total period of 9 weeks. Where cases were being treated conservatively no bracing or serious activity restriction was advised, and the child was assessed initially at 2 months and then at 3 monthly intervals until healing was established. From this time follow-up was performed on a 6 monthly basis. Standard radiographs taken in the antero-posterior and Lauenstein lateral views were obtained during the active phase of the disease. In 6 cases at-risk signs developed during conservative therapy, all these children were treated by operation.

Assessment

In all cases the disease was healed at the time of final assessment. The cases were assessed by Mr W. Muirhead-Allwood and given a 'good', 'fair' or 'poor' result using the criteria already discussed (Figs 9.3, 9.4, 9.5). This is the same assessment as that used by Lloyd-Roberts et al (1976) and Brotherton (1977) and therefore allows a comparison of these series of cases.

Results of treatment

Overall results

By comparison with untreated controls (Table 9.5) the overall results showed a reduced number of poor results and an increased percentage of those obtaining a good outcome (Table 9.6).

Table 9.5 Untreated cases

	No.	Good %	Fair %	Poor %
All cases	95	57	19	24
Groups II III IV	75	44	33	23
Groups II III IV at-risk	54	31	28	41

Table 9.6 Overall results.

	No.	Good %	Fair %	Poor %
All cases	89	64	21	15
Groups II III IV	72	56	26	18

Table 9.7 Early untreated cases.

Group	No.	Good	Fair	Poor
I	17	17	0	0
II	8	8	0	0
III	2	2	0	0
IV	3	1	0	2
Total	30	28 (93%)	0	2 (7%)

Table 9.8 Healing untreated cases.

Group	No.	Good	Fair	Poor
II	6	1	4	1
III	6	0	3	3
IV	7	1	2	4
Total	19	2 (11%)	9 (47%)	8 (42%)

Untreated cases

Of the 89 hips, 49 (55 per cent) had received no treatment (Tables 9.2, 9.5, 9.6). In 30 this was because of the absence of at-risk signs and in 19 healing was established and definitive treatment by operation considered ineffective. Of the 30 hips prospectively untreated during the active phase of the disease 28 obtained good results. Twenty-five of these were in Groups I and II. The poor results will be considered separately.

Fig. 9.1 A child aged 5 years with Group IV Legg-Calvé-Perthes' disease treated by femoral osteotomy.

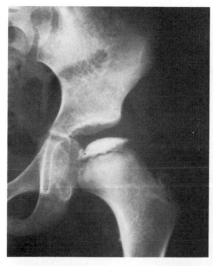

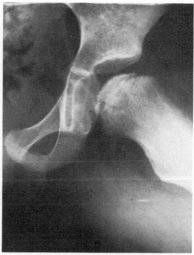

Fig. 9.1(a) July 1973. Antero-posterior and lateral radiographs of the left hip. There are changes compatible with Group IV disease, particularly on the lateral view where there is beaking of the posterior metaphysis. There is lateral uncovering and a horizontal growth plate.

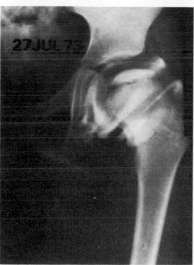

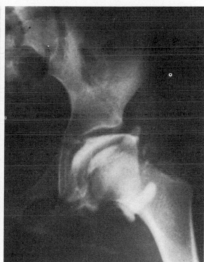

Fig. 9.1(b) The radiographs taken at the time of arthrography. These show on the left that the congruous position of this femoral head is in the position of 15 degrees of adduction. There is considerable uncovering of the femoral head, particularly of its lateral cartilagenous part. On the right the position of abduction and internal rotation showing containment of the femoral head within the mould of the acetabulum.

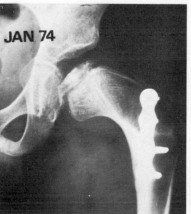

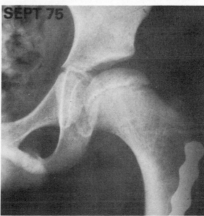

Fig. 9.1(c) Radiographs taken in January 1974 and September 1975. These show containment of the femoral head following osteotomy and a good result at the time of healing. The final radiograph in this case is Figure 9.3.

Fig. 9.2 Group III disease. A child with Group III disease aged 6 years 6 months treated by innominate osteotomy.

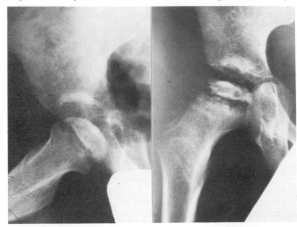

Fig. 9.2(a) April 1974. Antero-posterior and lateral radiographs showing Group III disease with a horizontal growth plate, a lytic area laterally (Gage's sign), a diffuse metaphyseal reaction and widening of the infero-medial joint space.

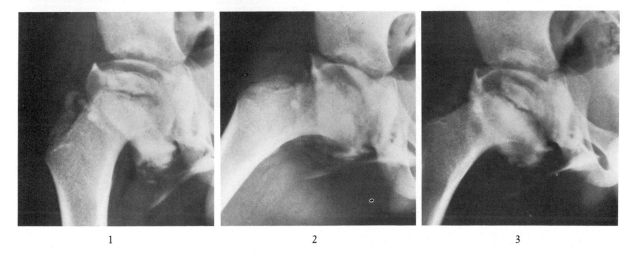

1   2   3

Fig. 9.2(b) August 1974. Radiographs obtained at the time of arthrography. Left (1) the neutral position, (2) in abduction and internal rotation, (3) in flexion, abduction and internal rotation. Best containment of the femoral head is in the position of flexion, abduction and internal rotation.

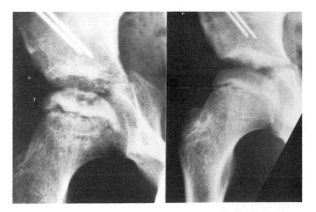

Fig. 9.2(c) Radiographs taken in August 1976 and August 1978, 2 and 4 years following innominate osteotomy showing reformation of the femoral head and containment within the acetabulum.

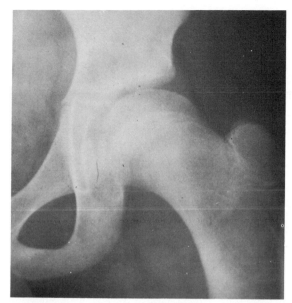

Fig. 9.3 A good result

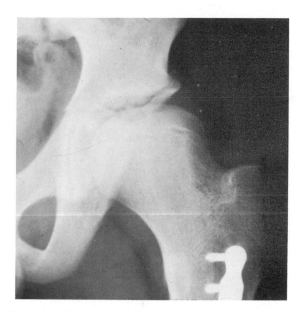

Fig. 9.4 A fair result.

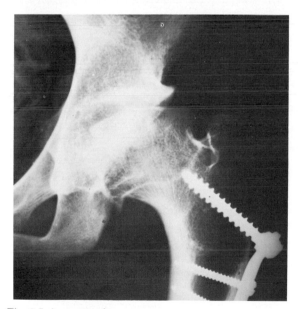

Fig. 9.5 A poor result.

Results of prospective treatment

It was felt important to separate those cases which were seen early in the disease process from those presenting late where the possible advantages of operative therapy were not available. When these were compared with the overall results and with untreated controls (Tables 9.5, 9.6 and 9.9) the incidence of a poor result can be seen to be reduced when the patient was cared for throughout the disease process and not just during the healing phase.

Table 9.9 Prospective results

Group	No.	Good	Fair	Poor
I	17	17	0	0
II	20	16 ⎫	3 ⎫	1 ⎫
III	23	15 ⎬72%	6 ⎬19%	2 ⎬9%
IV	10	7 ⎭	1 ⎭	2 ⎭
Total	70	55 (79%)	10 (14%)	5 (7%)

Operative treatment

Femoral and innominate osteotomy (Tables 9.5 and 9.10) improve the outcome when compared with untreated controls in Groups II, III and IV at-risk. Not only was there an increase in the incidence of a good result but a reduction in the poor results from 41 per cent to 8 per cent. The 3 poor results were all over the age of 8 years at the

Table 9.10 Osteotomy results

Group	No.	Good	Fair	Poor
II	12	8	3	1
III	21	13	6	2
IV	7	6	1	0
Total	40	27 (67%)	10 (25%)	3 (8%)

time of primary presentation. One of the important aspects of operative treatment was its ability to reverse the process of femoral head flattening (Fig. 9.1). This can be demonstrated by comparing the pre-operative arthrograms with the final result.

Age

As in previous reports the importance of age as a long term prognostic factor has been confirmed with a considerable reduction in the chance of a good result with disease starting over the age of 6 years (Table 9.11).

Table 9.11 Results related to age.

		No.	Good %	Fair %	Poor %
Under 6 years	Untreated controls	26	54	34	12
	Osteotomy	12	83	17	0
Over 6 years	Untreated controls	18	17	33	50
	Osteotomy	28	60	29	11

The Groups III and IV cases

It was felt important to consider the Groups' III and IV cases separately because of the number of poor results seen in these Groups. Also Brotherton and McKibbin (1977) have shown a striking difference in outcome for Group IV cases treated by prolonged recumbancy and femoral head containment. In the present series the overall results of the Group III cases do not seriously differ from those reported by Lloyd-Roberts (1976) and Brotherton and McKibbin (1977) except that in the present series 8 (27 per cent) of the 29 cases had received no treatment. In the Group IV cases although the numbers are small where adequate clinical control was maintained throughout the active phase there are no poor results. The fact that the 2 poor results in this prospective Group occurred when out-patient supervision was inadequate underlines the value of surgical treatment in the management of these cases. It also supports the indication for early operative treatment in the management of these

problems. Where possible it should be undertaken before deformity of the femoral head is present. The majority of the poor results in the Group IV Cases were in fact seen in those cases in which healing was present at the time of clinical presentation and for whom operative treatment was considered not to be beneficial (Table 9.8). In the light of these results however, it is to be questioned whether the presence of healing in the Group IV cases is necessarily a contraindication to treatment if the present treatment protocols are followed.

Conclusions

It is accepted that the number of cases presented in this study are too small for statistical comparisons to be made and it is therefore possible only to recognise trends, the proof of which will require a larger series of cases. This series of cases has been prospectively treated in order to test the hypothesis 'Will treatment only help selected cases?'. When comparison is made with previous reports the severity of disease, age and at-risk factors are similar as are the overall results. However, the essential difference between this series and other reports is that 55 per cent have received no treatment. This casts doubt on the effectiveness of many forms of treatment, particularly when the disease is in the healing phase. These results support the suggestion made by Lloyd-Roberts et al (1976) and Canario et al (1980) that the poor results following operation were seen in those children where the disease process was of more than 20 months duration. Of the 19 cases presenting during the healing phase 8 attained a poor result without treatment, 4 of which were in the Group IV cases. In view of the extremely good results reported by Brotherton and McKibbin (1977) for Group IV cases it is to be questioned whether even in the healing phases operative treatment should not be more seriously considered.

Where adequate clinical control was available during the early and active phases of the disease the results show a substantial improvement over the untreated controls. Of this prospective Group 30 (45 per cent) again received no treatment. Of these 17 were in Group I and all obtained a good result which could have been anticipated from the natural history of the process. The remaining cases had more severe involvement, of which 5 were in Groups III and IV. Three of these achieved a good result. In the final 2, through inadequate out-patient supervision, the indications for surgical treatment were not observed and the final result was poor. These results support the theory that surgical treatment can prevent serious deformity of the femoral head from occurring particularly when it is undertaken at an early stage.

The theories and principles upon which the indications for definitive and conservative treatment are based have been carefully tested in this series. It may be concluded that where there are no indications for definitive treatment, particularly during the early phases of the disease, management may be conservative in the first instance. Should at-risk signs appear during subsequent course of the disease the overall result does not seem to be prejudiced, provided treatment is promptly undertaken (Fig. 9.6). An analysis of the results does not lend support to the philosophy

Fig. 9.6 Child aged 5 years 6 months with Group III disease.

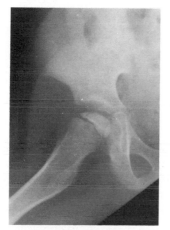 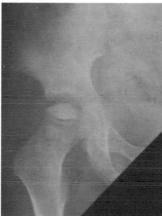

Fig. 9.6(a) September 1976. Antero-posterior and lateral views showing early lateral uncovering. Treatment was conservative.

Fig. 9.6(b) March 1977. There is now lateral uncovering, calcification lateral to the epiphysis and a horizontal growth plate. There is a reduced range of movement (signs at-risk).

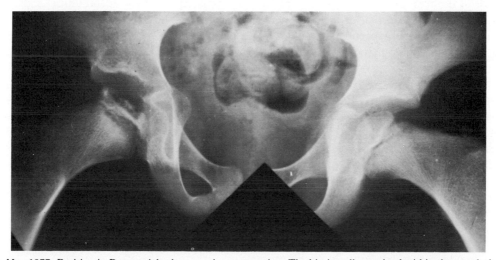

Fig. 9.6(c) May 1977. Position in Broomstick plasters prior to operation. The hip is well contained within the acetabulum and the hip has regained its mobility.

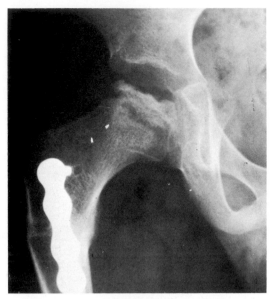

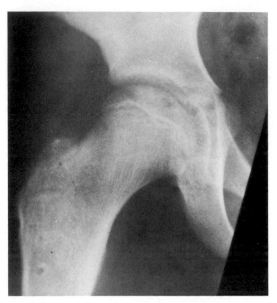

Fig. 9.6(d) August 1977. Following varus rotation osteotomy of the femur the hip remains well seated and is now in the healing phase.

Fig. 9.6(e) August 1980. The disease is healed with a good result.

that treatment, particularly by splintage, is indicated in the early phase of the condition before the definitive radiological signs of Group and at-risk become apparent.

The problem of weight relief requires further consideration. In both our prospective series and the cases reported by Brotherton and McKibbin (1977) the initial phases of treatment have common factors; the restoration of movement and containment of the femoral head within the mould of the acetabulum. Based on an understanding of the morbid anatomy it has been concluded that the major principle of treatment is the restoration of movement to permit normal growth and remodelling. It is suggested that this pre-operative mobilisation is important because it permits better containment of the femoral head, particularly with a better range of internal rotation. The subsequent femoral osteotomy is then more effective in producing containment of the femoral head. The evidence from the present series of cases, therefore, would challenge the concept of weight relief as the essential component of therapy for Group IV cases and suggests that where treatment is instituted in the active phase mobility of the hip in the contained position is the more essential factor. The series reported by Brotherton

and McKibbin (1977) utilised both this concept and that of weight relief to the same extent.

In the healing cases the important principle of long term congruency of the joint or congruous incongruity (Curtis 1978) would seem to be of importance. With a knowledge of the morphology in the healing phase two types of abnormality could be present, singularly or in combination. These are hinge abduction and disproportion between the femoral head and the acetabulum. The first can be reversed by abduction osteotomy (Fig. 8.9). If it is considered that the degree of disproportion between the femoral head and acetabulum is sufficient to cause symptoms in the patient then treatment by acetabular enlargement would seem to be indicated. The author has no experience of these latter procedures in this condition but the reported results of the Chiari operation and acetabuloplasty (Van der Heydon and Van Tongerloo 1980) would suggest that there may be a place for these procedures in the long term management.

REFERENCES

Brotherton B J, McKibbin B 1977 Perthes' disease treated by prolonged recumbancy and femoral head containment, a long term appraisal. Journal of Bone and Joint Surgery 59B: 14

Canario A T, Williams L, Wientroub S, Catterall A, Lloyd-Roberts G C 1980 A controlled study of the results of femoral osteotomy in severe Perthes' disease. Journal of Bone and Joint Surgery 62B: 438–440

Curtis B H 1978 Personal communication

Lloyd-Roberts G C, Catterall A, Salamon P B 1976 A controlled study of the indications and results of femoral osteotomy in Perthes' disease. Journal of Bone and Joint Surgery 58B: 31–36

Muirhead-Allwood M 1980 Personal communication

Van der Heyden A M, Van Tongerloo R B 1980 Shelf operation in Perthes' disease. Paper presented to Continental Meeting of Dutch, Norvic and British Orthopaedic Associations, October 1980.

10

The future

It must be the first conclusion of this book that the cause of Legg-Calvé-Perthes' disease remains unknown. However, the evidence presented in the various chapters does support the hypothesis that was set out in Chapter 1. This stated that:

> In the suscpetible child the changes which are called Legg-Calvé-Perthes' disease are the consequence of ischaemia of variable duration, after which the process of repair produces a growth disturbance, which if uncontrolled leads to femoral head deformity with subsequent arthritis.

The evidence has posed many questions to which answers will have to be found. These answers will in themselves support or reject the hypothesis.

The hypothesis does, however, suggest where our further industries should be directed. These efforts will have to be on several fronts: the susceptible child, the ischaemic process, the growth disturbance and its control, and the degenerative arthritis. At the present time the first three would seem to stimulate the most thought and therefore to suggest avenues of research which might profitably be examined.

By careful clinical examination, research and education it should be possible to define more precisely the susceptible child. Minor symptoms of hip disease in these children would permit an early diagnosis of this condition during the early active phase of the disease and before severe deformity of the femoral head had occurred. It has been suggested that treatment undertaken during this stage will be more profitable than that undertaken during the healing phase. This problem, therefore, should be one of the first aspects of this disease to be tackled.

At a clinical level the question of treatment will continue to merit much discussion. If subsequent reports using the protocols described confirm the results presented in this series, then it would seem to me that treatment can improve the outcome of selected cases where it is undertaken early in the active phase of the disease. However, much more research, possibly with a change in the principles of treatment, will be required in the management of the older child presenting during the healing phase of this condition with considerable deformity of the femoral head. Is it possible by reconstructive surgery at this stage to prevent the degenerative arthritis which we already know will be the long term outcome of this severely misshapen femoral head? A knowledge of these factors will allow proper indications for the major reconstructive procedures, such as the Chiari operation, acetabulaplasty and chielotomy. Also at a clinical level much more information is required on the endocrine status of these children. Growth is now known to be controlled by the complex interaction of a number of hormones. The fact that a particular hormone is either on the low or high side of normal may represent a major upset in this complex interaction and therefore the growth process. In this matter we are once again in the hands of the scientists but it must be clinical examination and judgement which suggest to these important research workers where possible lines of investigation will lie.

At a more fundamental level it has not been possible until the present time to reproduce in the experimental animal the changes seen in Legg-

Calvé-Perthes' disease in human. Even in those animals which are known to develop this process spontaneously, the underlying cause cannot be established. Although a number of workers have already pursued this problem it would seem that simple ischaemia will not in itself result in the changes seen in human material. It would appear necessary to interfere with the process of repair and considerable further research will be required into this problem before an experimental model can be reproduced.

With regard to the degenerative arthritis it is beyond the terms of reference of this presentation to consider how this may be treated. It is, however, the hope that with time, research and the acquisition of further knowledge, the surgery required for the late manifestions of this condition may be prevented by early treatment.

Index

Abduction osteotomy, 97
Acetabuloplasty, 97, 108
Acetabulum
  lateral lip, 68, 97
  potential for change, 86–88
  quotient, 86
  tear drop, 44
Adduction contracture, 36, 71, 77
Aetiology, 3–6
  constitutional factors, 3, 4
  skeletal age, 4, 5, 6
  skeletal maturation, 4
  stature, 4
Age, 34, 58, 81, 85
  of bone, 5, 6, 88
  within Groups, 58
  at healing, 65–67
  long term prognosis, 65–67
  maternal, 4
  onset, 34
  poor result, 67, 106
  results of operation in relation to, 106
Anteversion of femoral neck, 86–87
Arteries
  circumflex femoral, 10
  lateral epiphyseal, 31
  profunda, 10
  retinacular, 10
Arthrography, 86, 88–90, 103–104
  findings, 89
  hinge abduction, 73, 89, 97
  indication for operation, 103–104
  late case, 89, 97–99
  in osteochondritis dissecans, 61–63
  technique, 89–90
Articular cartilage
  anatomy of, 9
  calcification of, 12
  remodelling of, 32
  thickening, 11, 12, 14, 18, 28, 32
  uninvolved hip, 12
Aspiration of hip joint, 35
Assessment
  age and sex, 85
  clinical, 88
  end results, 84, 102
  factors, 84
  late cases, 97–99
  methods, 84
Avascular necrosis, 8, 31

Bed rest, 81, 82
Bilateral cases, 34, 40
  age, 34–35
  radiological signs, 40
  sex, 35
  sex ratio, 35
Biological remodelling, 77, 97
Birth weight, 4
Bone age, 5, 6, 88
Bone marrow
  calcification of, 15
  fatty replacement, 30
  necrosis of, 8, 11, 15
Bone necrosis, 8, 11, 13–26
Bone scan, 37
  cold spots, 37
  in healing disease, 37
  in irritable hip, 37
Bone trabeculae, 9
Broadening of femoral head, 74
Broomstick plaster, 92
  adjustable, 92, 102

Calcification lateral to epiphysis, 74
Calcification of articular cartilage, 12
Capsular shadow, 43
C.E. angle of Wiberg, 65, 87
Chiari operation, 97, 108, 110
Chielectomy, 97, 108, 110
Chondrification of the infarct, 28, 32
Clinical assessment, 88, 101
Clinical features
  age and sex, 34
  bilateral cases, 34
  examination, 36
  investigation, 37
  presentation, 35
Concept of head-at-risk, 76
Congenital anomalies, 5
Congenital heart disease, 5
Congruity, 32, 89
Congruous incongruity, 32, 69, 84, 108
Constitutional factors, 4, 5
Containment of femoral head, 81, 82, 83, 91
  maintenance of, 91–92
  by operation, 81, 82
  by splint, 81, 82

Contracture
  adduction, 36, 88
  flexion, 36, 88
Contra-indication to treatment, 86
  to operation, 5, 13
Core biopsy, 8, 12
Course of disease, 5, 14, 61
Coxa Magna, 35
Coxa Vara, 94
Creeping substitution, 8, 11, 18
Cretinism, 37

Degree of radiological involvement, 45–59
Dent on femoral head, 72, 73
Deterioration of head shape, 74–76
  radiological signs of deformity, 71–74, 83
Diagnosis — early, 34, 44, 110
Differential diagnosis
  irritable hip syndrome, 35
  Perthes-like change, 39
Double infarction, 8
Duration of disease, 60–61
  effect of osteotomy, 61
Duration of symptoms, 88

Early diagnosis, 34, 44, 110
Effective treatment, 70, 92
Endochondral ossification, 10, 13
End results, 81
Eosinophilic granuloma, 42
Epidemiological factors, 4
  length of gestation, 4
  parental age, 4
  parity, 4
  social class, 4
Epiphysis
  blood supply, 9
  broadening, 13
  calcification lateral to, 53, 74
  collapse of, 15, 18, 53, 84
  degree of involvement, 45–56
  density, 45
  height, 14, 86
  infarction of, 11, 18, 28, 32

Epiphysis (*contd*)
  ischaemia of, 9, 11
  normal anatomy, 9
  size, 45
  trabeculae, 9, 71
  uninvolved hip, 13
E.S.R., 37
Examination under anaesthetic, 88–90
Examination
  clinical, 36, 88
  follow-up, 37

Family history, 36
Femoral head
  blood supply, 9
  containment of, 82, 91
  deformity of, 67, 71–74, 83
  dent, 73
  lateral displacement, 44, 67
  osteochondritis dissecans, 61–63
  normal anatomy, 9
  plasticity of, 83
Femoral neck
  angle of, 87, 94
  anteversion, 86, 87
  differential ratio of growth, 74, 83
  quotient, 87
Femoral osteotomy, 32
  heat-at-risk, 80, 85, 102
  indication for, 80, 86, 102–104
  technique, 95–97
Fibrocartilagenous material, 27, 32
Fixed subluxation
  follow-up, 36
  fragmentation, 49
  Frog-lateral position, 39

Gage's sign, 74
Gait, 36
Gaucher's disease, 37, 40
General health, 36
Genetic factors, 4
Genito-urinary disease, 5, 6
Girls
  age of onset, 34
  bilateral cases, 34
  poor prognosis, 58
Granulation tissue, 11, 18
Groups, 45–59, 71, 77, 85, 106
  age and sex ratios, 58
  assessment of radiological signs, 47
  course of the disease, 47–49, 53–54
  epiphyseal signs, 47
  femoral osteotomy, 9, 94–95
  Group I, 47
  Group II, 48–49
  Group III, 49–53, 106
  Group IV, 53–57, 106
  histological appearances, 13–28
  indications for treatment, 82, 85, 86
  metaphyseal signs, 47
  results in untreated cases, 57, 77

Image intensifier, 89
Incidence
  in families, 3
  Merseyside, 3
  rural areas, 3
  Scotland, 3
  towns, 3
  world figures, 3
Indications for treatment, 84
  abduction osteotomy, 89, 108
  conservative, 86, 102
  definitive, 102
  femoral osteotomy, 89
  for I.V.P., 5, 37, 47
  Groups, 86
  head-at-risk, 74, 80, 85, 86
  innominate osteotomy, 89
  in long term, 70
Infarction of epiphysis, 18, 71
  consequence of, 11
  extent of, 18
  incomplete, 17
  repeated, 28
  single episode, 9, 32
  total, 28
  two episodes, 8, 32
Infection, 40
Inguinal hernia, 4, 88
Inherited factors, 3
Intra-epiphyseal gas, 44
Investigation, 37
Irritable hip syndrome, 35, 44
  differential diagnosis, 35–36
  long term results, 35
Ischaemia of variable duration, 2, 31, 110
Islands of cartilage, 32
I.V.P. indications for, 5, 37

Joint contracture, 71, 72, 73
Joint space
  infero-medial, 44
Juvenile rheumatoid arthritis, 36

Kohler's disease, 36

Late cases, 89, 97
Lateral displacement of the femoral head, 44, 89, 97
Lateral radiographs, 39
Lateral subluxation, 76, 77
  measurement of, 76
Lateral uncovering, 67
Lauenstein position, 39, 44, 47
Length of gestation, 4
Limp, 36, 88
Long term prognosis, 65–80
  age at time of healing, 67
  irregular femoral head, 65, 78
  lateral subluxation, 76
  poor result in long term, 79

premature growth plate arrest, 68
  radiological changes, 69
Loose body, 61–63
Loss of epiphyseal height, 14, 86
Lymphoma, 37, 40
  lytic defects, 47

Neck length ratio, 60
Necrosis
  avascular, 8, 31
  of bone, 3, 8, 11, 13–26
  marrow, 8, 14, 15

Maintenance of containment, 92–95
Marrow
  calcification of, 15
  fatty replacement, 30
  necrosis, 8, 14
Measurements
  E.A., 65
  neck length, 60
  of quotients, 65, 86–88
  of subluxation, 76
Mechanism of femoral head deformity, 71–74
  radiological signs, 74
Metaphyseal changes, 28, 48, 53, 59
  fatty replacement, 30
  head-at-risk, 75, 77
  histological appearances, 28–31
  radiological, diffuse, 47, 59–60, 75
    localised, 47, 60, 75
Metaphysis, 40
  within femoral head, 9
Methods of treatment, 83, 101
  by operation, 94
  by splints, 93
Morbid anatomy, 8–33
Mose radius, 86
Movements of hip, 88
  normal, 83
  restoration of, 83, 108
Multiple epiphyseal dysplasia, 36, 37, 40
Myxoedema, 37, 40

Onset of symptoms, 35 88
Operative treatment, 94
Orthotic treatment, 92–93
  cessation of, 93
Osteoarthritis, 65, 69
Osteochondritis, 8
Osteochondritis dissecans, 61–63
  incidence, 61
  loose body, 61, 97
Osteotomy
  abduction, 97, 105
  acetabuloplasty, 97, 108, 110
  advantages, 94
  Chiari, 97, 108, 110
  chielectomy, 97, 108, 110

disadvantages, 94
femoral, 84, 89, 102
innominate, 89 102
technique of femoral, 95–97
trochanteric epiphysiodesis, 97

Pain in the hip, 36
Pain in the knee, 36
Parental age, 4
Parity, 4
Past and present, 1
Pendulum of change, 81
Perichondral ring, 12
Perthes-like change, 37
  differential diagnosis, 37
Poor result, 57, 71–80
  long term, 79
Potential for remaining growth, 86–88
Premature arrest of growth plate, 67, 68
  complete, 68
  partial, 68
Presentation
  acute, 35
  chronic, 36
Prevention of ischaemia, 83
Principles of treatment, 82
  new, 83
  old, 82
  prevention of ischaemia, 83–84
  restoration of movement, 83
Process of repair, 8, 31
Pyloric stenosis, 5

Quotients
  acetabular, 86–88
  C.E. angle, 87
  epiphyseal, 87
  femoral, 87

Radiological signs of deterioration in
      head shape, 74–76
  broadening of epiphysis, 74
  calcification lateral to epiphysis, 74
  diffuse metaphyseal change, 75
  Gage's sign, 74
  lateral subluxation, 76
Range of movement, 71
Rates of growth
  femur, 6
  tibia, 6
Recurrent ischaemia, 83
Relief of weight, 82, 83, 108
Repair, process of, 31

Restoration of movement, 83, 108
  Broomstick plaster, 92
Results
  fair, 57, 79, 102
  good, 57, 79, 102
  healing, 102
  of operation, 105
  overall, 102
  poor, 57, 79, 102
  prospective, 101–108
  in relation to age, 58
  untreated cases, 57, 102
Review
  1970, 5, 65
  1980, 101

Sagging rope sign, 69
Sclerosis
  epiphyseal, 14, 45
Sequestrum, 47, 48, 49, 53
Sex, 34, 58, 59, 81, 84, 85
  bilateral cases, 34
  ratio, 34, 59
Shenton's line, 71
Shortening, 97
Short stature, 4
Sickle cell disease, 40
Signs
  of deterioration of shape of femoral
          head, 74–76
  Gage's, 74
  of head-at-risk, 77, 85
  of healing, 61, 85
  Sagging rope sign, 69
  'V' sign, 48
Skeletal age, 5, 6, 88
Skeletal maturation, 5, 6
Slipped epiphysis, 37
Social class, 4
Splints, 81
  containment, 81
  mobile, 81
  weight relieving, 81
Spondylo-epiphyseal dysplasia, 40
Stage of disease at diagnosis, 45, 81, 84
Stiffness
  head-at-risk, 77
  of subtaloid joint, 36
Still's disease, 36
Subchondral fracture line, 44, 48, 49, 53
Subluxation, 73
  fixed, 76
  index, 76
  lateral, 76, 77
  measurement of, 76
Subtaloid joint, 36

Tamponade theory, 11, 31
Tear drop, 44
Theory
  positional, 31
  Tamponade, 11, 31
Thomas' test, 36
Thyroid disorders, 4
Trabeculae
  crushing of, 15, 17, 18, 32, 71
  fracture of, 18
  in normal femoral head, 9
  remodelling of, 15, 28
  resorption of avascular, 11
Traction, 81
Transient synovitis of hip, 35
Treatment
  bed rest and traction, 81
  containment, 83
  contra-indications, 86
  early cases, 92
  femoral osteotomy, 81, 94
  Group III/IV, 106
  indication, 84–86
  innominate osteotomy, 81, 94
  late cases, 7, 97–99
  non operative, 81, 93
  operation, 81, 94
  principles, 82
  weight relieving methods, 81, 82
Trochanter
  overgrowth, 94
  epiphysiodesis of, 97

Uncovering of the femoral head, 73
Undescended testicle, 4, 36
Unilateral cases, 40
  controls, 57
  duration of disease, 60, 61
  late cases, 97
  neck ratio, 60
Uninvolved hips, 12, 86–88
Urinary infection, 45

Varus osteotomy, 84, 87
Vastus lateralis, 95
'V' sign, 48

Wasting of muscles, 44
Weight
  relief of, 82, 83, 108